BESTSELLING AUTHOR OF *A NEW NAME*

Emma Scrivener

A New Day

'A remarkable
and unique book'
Mark Meynell

Moving on from
hunger, anxiety,
control, shame,
anger and despair

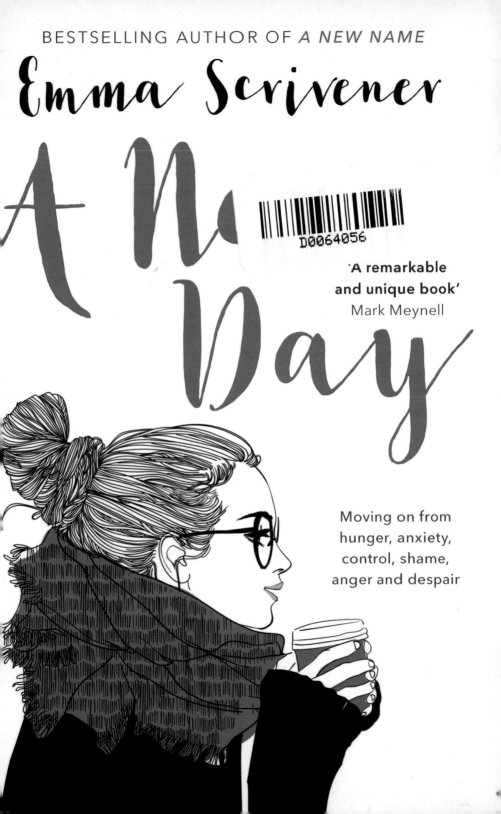

Our churches are full of hurting people, because they are full of ordinary men and women. Sometimes it is hard to share, especially if the issues are emotional or concerned with mental health. But the gospel speaks to the whole person, body, mind, emotions and spirit. In this book, Emma writes for those who are struggling and those who care for them. She writes not as an ivory-tower theorist, but as someone who has fought her own battles with God's help. Taking a helpful model of moving from darkness into light, she is real about human experience, but confident in Jesus' ability to enter into our struggles with his healing and redeeming power. This is a book that is both realistic and hopeful, linking experience to the gospel, so that life may be lived, moving from darkness into light.

Richard Jackson, Bishop of Lewes

What if mental health issues are not the problem of an unfortunate but limited few? What if everyone struggles? And what if there is a way forward? This is not just a book to help you understand others and help them, although it is that. This is a book to help you understand yourself, and even more importantly, to point you to the hope offered by Jesus Christ. Jesus is the one who enters into our mess, and it is when we meet him that we find hope – not an instant fix, but real hope. Whether you've known Jesus for years or are yet to meet him, let Emma Scrivener point you to Christ. This book will lift your heart as you struggle, and guide you practically as you reach out to help others. May it not only help individuals, but also stir whole churches to become communities of care, help and hope.

Peter Mead, Director of Cor Deo, author and Pastor, Trinity Church, Chippenham

This is a remarkable and unique book which deserves a wide reader-ship. Emma Scrivener has shown great courage yet again in writing about her own pain and brokenness in order to speak into a huge range of personal crises, but she does so with creativity, deep pastoral sensitivity and clear gospel convictions. This is that rare book that can truly speak into the darkness of our pain without any judgments at the same time as holding out the genuine hope of lasting change.

Mark Meynell, Associate Director, Langham Partnership

This is a disarming book. If you have anorexia, it could help save your life; even if you don't, it will touch your life in one area or another because we are all made of the same clay as Emma; it's just that some are better at hiding their frailties than others. The deliberate exposure of one's own vulnerability can be a powerful therapeutic tool in its own right, but when accompanied by such a wealth of practical advice, checklists, case studies and resources as here, it ensures this book will help thousands of readers to cherish their bodies as God intends.
Trevor Stammers, Senior Lecturer in Bioethics, St Mary's University, London, and Editor, The New Bioethics

It's easy to feel alone when we're struggling. It's common to feel confused when we're supporting friends. That's why it is so valuable to have short books like this that put voice to people's pain and hope in people's hearts. Written in Emma's usual engaging style, and drawing on a wealth of real-life conversations, *A New Day* takes a walk through the experience of emotional pain and shows that the gospel has something powerful to say to Christians and non-Christians alike. Her humility, gentleness and confidence in the Lord weave through every page as she encourages fellow strugglers to move from darkness to light. And, while there is much more that can be said about complex issues such as these, if you are looking for an accessible place to begin, there is a great deal to commend this short resource.
Helen Thorne, Director of Training and Mentoring, London City Mission

I am convinced this profound book needs to be read in little bites. Emma Scrivener shares her scars as she pulls back the curtain on hunger, anxiety, control, shame, anger and despair. And if we groan 'Me too', then we need to take time not only to see our chains, but also to rejoice in the real, grounded, hard-won, tear-stained, Christ-centred answers Emma wonderfully holds out to us.
Rico Tice, Associate Minister, All Souls, Langham Place, London

Emma writes with beautiful and striking honesty, having known for herself the reality of Jesus in the midst of a very dark night. Anyone would find help from this trustworthy book, which shows the ability of the gospel to connect gloriously with raw life, pain and need.
Joel Virgo, Senior Pastor, Church of Christ the King, Brighton

A New Day

Emma Scrivener

A New

Day

Moving on from hunger, anxiety,
control, shame, anger and despair

Emma Scrivener

INTER-VARSITY PRESS
36 Causton Street, London SW1P 4ST, England
Email: ivp@ivpbooks.com
Website: www.ivpbooks.com

© Emma Scrivener, 2017

Emma Scrivener has asserted her right under the Copyright, Designs and Patents Act 1988 to be identified as Author of this work. All rights reserved. No part of this publication may be reproduced, stored in a retrieval system, or transmitted, in any form or by any means, electronic, mechanical, photocopying, recording or otherwise, without the prior permission of the publisher or the Copyright Licensing Agency.

Unless otherwise indicated, Scripture quotations are taken from the Holy Bible, New International Version (Anglicized edition). Copyright © 1979, 1984, 2011 by Biblica (formerly International Bible Society). Used by permission of Hodder & Stoughton Publishers, an Hachette UK company. All rights reserved. 'NIV' is a registered trademark of Biblica (formerly International Bible Society). UK trademark number 1448790.

Scripture quotations marked NLT are taken from the Holy Bible, New Living Translation, copyright © 1996, 2004, 2007 by Tyndale House Foundation. Used by permission of Tyndale House Publishers, Inc., Carol Stream, Illinois 60188. All rights reserved.

The Scripture quotation marked AMP is from the Amplified Bible. Copyright © 2015 by The Lockman Foundation, La Habra, CA 90631. All rights reserved.

The Scripture quotation marked NASB is taken from the NEW AMERICAN STANDARD BIBLE®, Copyright © 1960, 1962, 1963, 1968, 1971, 1972, 1973, 1975, 1977, 1995 by The Lockman Foundation. Used by permission.

The Scripture quotation marked KJV is taken from the Authorized Version of the Bible (The King James Bible), the rights in which are vested in the Crown, and is reproduced by permission of the Crown's Patentee, Cambridge University Press.

First published 2017

British Library Cataloguing-in-Publication Data
A catalogue record for this book is available from the British Library.

ISBN: 978–1–78359–441–2
eBook ISBN: 978–1–78359–531–0

Set in Chapperal 12/15pt
Typeset in Great Britain by CRB Associates, Potterhanworth, Lincolnshire
Printed in Great Britain by Ashford Colour Press Ltd, Gosport, Hampshire

Inter-Varsity Press publishes Christian books that are true to the Bible and that communicate the gospel, develop discipleship and strengthen the church for its mission in the world.

IVP originated within the Inter-Varsity Fellowship, now the Universities and Colleges Christian Fellowship, a student movement connecting Christian Unions in universities and colleges throughout Great Britain, and a member movement of the International Fellowship of Evangelical Students. Website: www.uccf.org.uk. That historic association is maintained, and all senior IVP staff and committee members subscribe to the UCCF Basis of Faith.

For my daughter

Contents

Acknowledgments

An enormous thank-you to everyone who has helped me with this book: my blog readers (for sharing their stories), Eleanor (for her wisdom and patience), Mum and Dad, Alan W., Judy, my servant-hearted church family and praying friends. Most of all, to Glen for carrying me to Jesus.

Introduction
A new start?

When I became a Christian I was told 'everything would change'. It did – but not quite as I'd expected.

Jesus was meant to save my life. I felt like he'd ruined it.

I was still bullied at school. I felt as lost and confused as ever, sometimes more. My family relationships broke down. My grandfather died, and I developed a life-threatening eating disorder along with depression and OCD.

The old me was sinful, but at least she made sense. She knew where she belonged and she slotted into place. The new me stuck out. She looked nothing like the speakers who came to our youth group:

'I was a drug addict and Jesus made me clean.'
'I had a stutter and now I can speak.'
'I was bullied but now I've got friends.'

These Christians seemed perfect. They didn't have problems, especially not with mental health. They didn't feel sad and hungry and angry and anxious and afraid. They trusted Jesus and he took their problems away.

But I trusted Jesus and he didn't take them away. I trusted Jesus and I was a mess.

I told myself to give it time. A few months, at least. *When you're fifteen, you'll be better. When you're twenty, you'll be fixed.* Each year I waited for the change I expected. Twenty-seven, twenty-nine, thirty, thirty-five.

Thirty-eight – and I'm still waiting. I still don't look like those Christians at youth group.

God is changing me, but I still have struggles with my mental health. I get anxious and depressed. I'm frightened of having needs. I try to be perfect and to do all things 'right'. I'd rather be comfortable than brave. I'm controlling and insecure and desperate to prove my own worth. I'm a Christian, but I don't always feel like it.

And I'm not alone. Throughout this book you'll see quotations in italics from courageous blog readers and friends; real-life stories and experiences like these:

Right now, I feel useless and worthless. I feel unclean and shameful. I feel guilty and an embarrassment. I feel like a failure, like I can get nothing right. I feel hatred towards myself because I do the things I do not want to do and do not do what I know I should do. I feel unlovable and messy. I feel broken and vulnerable and fragile and weak. I feel marred and sinful. I feel lonely and isolated. I feel anxious and scared. I feel ugly. I feel sad and hurt. I feel angry and resentful and bitter. I feel damaged and tainted. I know these things are not true, but right now that's how I feel.

Can you identify with these words? I can. Churches are full of hurting people, but as we'll see, they can also be places of healing and hope. However, even in church some problems can be more acceptable than others.

If I break my arm, friends rally round. They ask how it happened, sympathize and provide practical support. There's a set time for recovery, and it's patently obvious what's wrong. No-one tells me to think myself better or have more faith. But if I'm struggling with mental health issues, that's not always the case. When we're self-harming or depressed, we can keep these things hidden. Treatment isn't straightforward, and there's no guarantee we'll be fixed. Other Christians can be wonderful, but occasionally they make judgments: 'If you prayed more, you wouldn't feel so anxious. If you had more faith, you wouldn't be stuck.' When we hear words like these, we tell ourselves, *I'm too much for God and the church. I'm too broken to change. I'm too tired to move forward . . .*

But what if . . .

. . . We're not alone?

What if everyone struggles? And what if, whatever we're facing or wherever we've been, we can all make a new start?

That's what *A New Day* is all about. It's written for struggling Christians and those who love them. And it offers hope to anyone who's ever felt too broken, too messy or too much.

Light for those in the dark

When I was small, I was scared of the dark. Mum would tuck me up into bed and turn on a nightlight, so I didn't feel so alone. It was a tiny lamp but it was enough to make me feel safe. It reminded me that morning was coming and the darkness would pass.

In some ways I'm still scared of the dark. Not the darkness outside, but the darkness inside me. This takes different forms: anxieties that quickly spiral into panic; a burning desire to be in control; anger that sparks from nothing and blazes into shame; doubts and hungers that I'm frightened to express. During the day I keep them at bay. But at night they won't be silenced.

If you can understand these feelings, then this book is for you. We'll be thinking specifically about mental health, but it's for everyone who's ever felt frightened or ashamed or angry or messy or alone. These things keep us in the dark, but the gospel offers us a way out. It points us to a God who illuminates the whole world and brings us into a community of light.

Around the clock

For the next twenty-four hours we'll be travelling together from darkness into light. Our day starts with night instead of morning, which might sound strange. But in the Bible the darkness comes first: 'And there was evening, and there was morning – the first day' (Genesis 1:5).

As we'll see, this is also a little picture of the Christian life.

Our day together is divided into two parts, moving from darkness (Part 1) into light (Part 2).

In Part 1 we'll think about our shared struggles (or 'darkness') and the ways we try to manage them (evening). Then we'll see how Jesus enters our suffering (midnight),

Our timetable

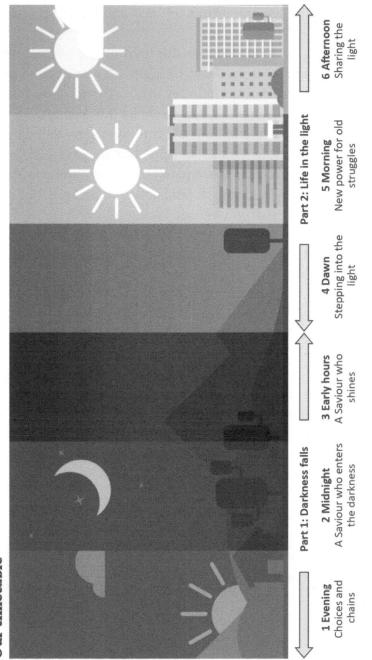

1 Evening
Choices and chains

Part 1: Darkness falls

2 Midnight
A Saviour who enters the darkness

3 Early hours
A Saviour who shines

4 Dawn
Stepping into the light

Part 2: Life in the light

5 Morning
New power for old struggles

6 Afternoon
Sharing the light

and finally how he brings us help and 'light' (the early hours).

Part 2 is about living in the light of the gospel. We'll look at how knowing Jesus changes our identity and self-image (dawn), how he helps us in our struggles (morning) and how we can help others in theirs (afternoon).

Throughout the book you'll find questions to help you think further, as well as an Appendix on page 175, with advice on specific issues and where to get more support.

At points you might be tempted to skip ahead, but let's stay together! If you're not facing all of the issues we cover, you can be sure someone close to you will be. And if they do apply to you, then be encouraged. By midday tomorrow we'll see:

Why we're broken – and how to be whole
Why we're stuck in the dark – and how we get out
Why we listen to lies – and how we fight back
What change looks like (and it's not what you'd guess)
How to resist anger, anxiety and despair
The difference between grief, guilt and shame
The place of professionals, pills and pastors
How to deal with regret
How and why our wounds can help to heal others
Why we're never alone in the dark – and how,
    together, we shine.

So let's start with evening, and the battles that *all* of us face.

Part 1

DARKNESS FALLS

1 Evening
Choices and chains

Imagine that we're at a dinner party and have just been introduced. As the wine is poured, we relax into our chairs and exchange pleasantries. *How was your journey? Have you come far?* Outside the wind is gathering and our host draws the curtains. After a moment I lean forward and smile: 'Tell me a bit about yourself.'

'Well,' you respond, 'I live near the seaside. I've got two kids, I work in the city and I like cinema and sports. How about you?'

I pause for a moment and set down my glass. 'Me?' I say. 'I'm hungry and I'm anxious. I'm controlling. I'm ashamed. I'm angry and I'm despairing. And I hope you don't mind me saying so – but I could see straight away, you're exactly the same.'

How do you react? Perhaps you're taken aback by my frankness. You wonder if I'm joking or exaggerating. You think to yourself, 'That's a lot of issues. This girl needs help.'

But maybe you're also slightly offended. 'Well,' you reply. 'Sometimes I lose my temper and I have days when it all feels a bit much. But I wouldn't put it like that. Angry and controlling? Surely that's a bit extreme?'

If our roles were reversed, I'd say the same thing. Hungry, anxious, ashamed, despairing? These are strong words – and we've only just met. But what if they came from the person who knows you best?

What if they came from God himself?

Well, let's prepare ourselves. Because this is what he says to us.

God created us and he knows us inside out. We're told this in the first book of the Bible (Genesis), where we also meet the first man and woman. Think of this couple as a picture of what it means to be human. Their problems are our problems, and their choices are the ones that we make too. Therefore, as we think about our own struggles, we're going to start with theirs. We'll see that they are *hungry* for life on their own terms, and so they become *anxious* about whether or not they'll be filled. They try to take *control* by disobeying God and are then burdened by *shame*. *Angrily* they turn on each other and they are then driven east of Eden in *despair*. That's their story in a nutshell, but it's our story too.

We're going to zoom in on the six particular issues: hunger, anxiety, control, shame, anger and despair. We'll look at how they shape the ways that we think and behave, both in healthy and unhealthy ways. At the end of each section you'll find a short list of questions to help you apply what you've been reading ('Thinking it through'). You can do these alone or with a friend. You might also use them as a starting point to talk to someone else,

	Hunger	Anxiety	Control	Shame	Anger	Despair
Adam and Eve	Wanting the fruit	Mistrusting God	Taking the fruit	Feeling naked	Blaming each other and lashing out	Driven out of Eden
Me	Wanting more than I have	Scared God won't provide for me	Taking charge of my life	Feeling exposed and ashamed	Frustrated with others and myself	Disappointed in others and myself
Examples	Eating disorders	Anxiety attacks	OCD	Self-harm	Aggression	Depression

especially if some of our topics touch on painful areas.
Also see 'Further help' on page 186.
   An outline is shown on page 5.
   Now let's begin.

Hunger

> Born ever-hungry,
> Hating our need.
> Despising dependence,
> Demanding our feed.
> Starving, stuffing,
> All or nothing.
> Since Adam and Eve
> We cannot receive.[1]

Glen and I have a daughter called Ruby who needs a
constant supply of food. Here's a typical day: 7 a.m.,
breakfast. Mid-morning, another snack. Brunch. Elev-
enses. Lunch. A mid-afternoon filler. Dinner, and then
supper. We always follow the same routine, and she's
learned to depend upon us, yet when she's hungry, she still
panics. Her eyes fill up, her face darkens and she howls as
though the world is ending. She tries to feed herself, but
not always wisely! In fact, she'll put anything in her mouth,
even if it causes her harm.

   This desperation is something that I can understand.

> Hunger is something that I've always felt. Not just for
> food – but for everything: from money to recognition.
> 'More!' is the cry of my heart. 'Give me more.' The emptier
> I feel, the more I need . . . and I'll do whatever it takes

to slake that thirst. Overworking. Overexercising. Overdrinking. Overspending. Overcleaning. There's just one problem. Whatever the fuel – clothes, booze, thinness – 'more' is never enough.[2]

I tried to fill my hungers with all sorts of 'food', from shopping to alcohol, exercise to work. When I bought four pairs of shoes, I was eating. When I exercised and drank and worked, I was trying to fill a hole. Yet whatever I tried, I still felt empty. So I went to the opposite extreme. Instead of trying to stuff myself, I starved. I became anorexic.

My eating disorder was never about feeling 'fat' (at least in the traditional sense). I didn't aspire to be a model and I didn't want to improve my appearance. 'Fat' was a description of all of my mess. It was all of the ways I stuck out at home and at school. It was my anger and fear and insecurity and sadness. It was the questions I had about life and death. It was the girl who was bullied and didn't fit in. These pressures made me feel like red wine spilt over a white cloth. By starving myself, I felt like I was mopping myself up:

By starving myself, I made myself clean. Instead of having lots of worries I couldn't manage, life became very simple. Controllable. With my body, I was able to create my own universe. A realm where I ruled, with unquestioned sovereignty. I was no longer at the mercy of my feelings. I was in charge: a self-created, stainless-steel person.[3]

Anorexia nearly destroyed me, but it felt like a solution. It gave me a sense of power, security and control. It was a way of handling my hungers and ruling my own world. The word 'anorexia' means loss of appetite, but nothing could be further from the truth. I was dominated by hunger – for affirmation, acceptance, purpose, identity and a million things I couldn't express. By starving myself, I silenced these hungers. I crushed them and I crushed them, until there was nothing left. No more feelings and no more 'fat'.

To those on the outside, eating disorders often appear baffling and extreme. Carers talk about feeling angry, confused, helpless and afraid. But they're responses to something equally threatening – our hungers.

Think for a moment about the things that you need: air, water, shelter, affection, love, security and relationships. They come from outside of us. They're a reminder that *we are not enough*. When we're hungry, we're scared that these needs won't be met, and so we cope by trying to feed ourselves. Some of us use food and some use work or sex or success; some of us stuff and some of us starve. Whatever our tactics, we're all trying to fill the same hole.

We see hunger as a curse, yet shockingly, God intended it as a blessing! To see why, let's go back to creation.

Imagine a luscious garden paradise, humming with colour and light. This is Eden, where God places the first man and woman. However, he doesn't leave them to fend for themselves. He shares his kingdom (Genesis 1:28–29), walks with them (3:8) and cherishes them as his children. Like a Father, he provides all that they need.

We do the same thing with our children, don't we? We feed them and we care for them. We walk with them and we guard them from harm. 'Don't play near the traffic,' we say. 'Stay away from the flames – or you'll be burned.'

Sometimes, however, our kids don't understand. Ruby is a good example. When I tell her that she can't have something, she wants it straight away: the jagged rock, the rusty tin opener, the kitchen cleaner, the kettle. In the course of the day we lurch from one potential disaster to another:

'Don't put your fingers in the plug socket.'

'Give the knife to Mummy.'

'What's that in your mouth? Spit it out, Ruby. Spit it out.'

When she points to the boiling potatoes, I shake my head. When she crawls towards the blender, I stand in her way.

'No,' I tell her. 'No' and 'no' and 'no' again. I carry her into another room, filled with toys. 'Ruby,' I say, 'Everything that I own is yours. But if you touch the blender, you'll cut your fingers. I know you want it. I'm saying no because I love you and I want to keep you safe.'

My words make no difference; she wants what she wants and she'll fight me to get it.

Something similar happens in the Garden of Eden.

Hunger in the garden

When God puts Adam and Eve in the garden, he gives them every tree but one. Just as I warn Ruby about the blender, he says, 'You are free to eat from any tree in the garden, but you must not eat from the tree of the knowledge of good and evil, for when you eat from it you will certainly die' (Genesis 2:16–17).

Adam and Eve refuse to obey. They ignore their real Father and instead they listen to the devil (the father of lies):

'You won't die!' the serpent [said] to the woman.

'God knows that your eyes will be opened as soon as

you eat it, and you will be like God, knowing both good and evil.'

The woman was convinced. She saw that the tree was beautiful and its fruit looked delicious, and she wanted the wisdom it would give her. So she took some of the fruit and ate it. Then she gave some to her husband, who was with her, and he ate it, too.
(Genesis 3:4–6, NLT)

This is much more serious than scrumping some fruit. In disobeying God, they reject him as their Father. They want to be *like* him and to take his place (see verse 5).

'Well,' we might argue, 'that's a nice story, but what's it got to do with me?' Answer: everything – according to the Bible. We live in the shadow of Adam and Eve's choices and we follow their example. We don't trust God either and we want to take his place. Instead of receiving from God, we rebel against him. 'We're hungry,' we say, 'But we'll provide for ourselves!'

The right kind of hunger

Hunger might feel threatening, but it can also be a gift. It shows our need for spiritual as well as physical food (Deuteronomy 8:3), and reminds us that God supplies both. Like an enormous neon arrow, it points to our Creator – but if we won't rely on him, the arrow points back to us. So we try to 'fill' ourselves. Perhaps we look to alcohol or self-medicate; perhaps we chase approval to boost our self-esteem. Perhaps we worry or throw ourselves into work. These are all ways of 'eating', but they leave us hungrier than before. They're like filling up on candyfloss, when what we really need is a good meal.

Thinking it through

In what ways do I use food to meet my emotional
needs?
Where do I look to be filled? Do these things satisfy?
Or are they more like 'junk food' – leaving me
wanting more?
How do I 'starve' (manage my needs through
self-denial) and 'stuff' (look to people or things
to make me feel full)?
Am I scared that God won't meet my needs?
What would it look like for me to give my hungers
to him?

Hunger at the extreme: eating disorders (EDs)
Eating disorders are ways of meeting emotional hungers
and using food to cope with life. By restricting food, we
feel in control. By overeating, we're sedating our fears.
By exercising or making ourselves sick, we're eliminating
our pain.

Who?
EDs affect around 1.6 million people in Britain, and
14–25-year-olds are most at risk. However, these figures
are often based on registered in-patients and exclude
those who have not come forward, are receiving private
treatment or are being treated as outpatients or in the
community.

• It's estimated that 10% of sufferers are anorexic,
40% are bulimic, and the rest are EDNOS
(see over).

- 5% of anorexia cases are fatal – making anorexia the deadliest mental illness.
- All sorts of people are affected: men (between 11% and 25%), women, children, seniors and Christians.[4]

What?

Anorexia nervosa: Restricting food intake (sometimes combined with excessive exercise).

Bulimia nervosa: Eating large quantities of food, then getting rid of it ('purging'), for example, by vomiting, abusing laxatives or exercising to excess.

Binge-eating disorder (BED): Bingeing on large quantities of food (see above) – but without purging.

Eating disorder not otherwise specified (EDNOS): This refers to eating disorders that don't meet the criteria for anorexia nervosa or bulimia nervosa (e.g. a woman who is anorexic, but still menstruating). It's the most common hospital diagnosis and a reminder that eating disorders don't fit into neat boxes. In fact, EDNOS can be especially distressing, as sufferers can feel they don't have a 'proper' diagnosis.

My anorexia began when I was forty-seven. It really began as I felt out of control with things in my life. I had gone back into the past to deal with childhood issues. I was under pressure at work, and working long hours, had elderly in-laws and a mum who was infirm. I began walking with friends and . . . found something I was good at. An inner voice took over, took control,

> *and I created rules about restricting food . . . I was admitted*
> *(for in-patient treatment) for several months. I came out*
> *having gained weight but not having addressed the issues*
> *of worthlessness, low self-esteem, perfectionism, etc. I am*
> *recovering, but I am not yet recovered.*

Summary

God made us to have hungers, but we reject him and try to feed ourselves. When we do, we're left empty and unsatisfied. This can lead to anxiety: our second issue.

Anxiety

When do you feel most anxious? For me it's sitting in the doctor's waiting room, opening test results, preparing for a difficult conversation or tackling a new project. At these points we tell ourselves, 'It'll all be OK.' We talk, pray and try to take hold of our worries. But sometimes our worries take hold of *us*.

> *Most of the time I'm not sure what I'm worrying about. I just*
> *feel nervous, uptight, sometimes physically in pain. I find*
> *it difficult to breathe . . . but as I don't know what's wrong,*
> *I never know what to do.*

The first time I had a panic attack, I had no idea what was happening. My heart was hammering, and I wanted to scream, but I could barely breathe. In fact, I thought that I was dying. One minute I felt fine, the next I was hunched over the pavement, gripped by an inexplicable fear. For weeks afterwards I stayed in my room, convinced that if I went out I'd have another attack. But withdrawing from others only made my anxiety worse. One worry spiralled into another, until everything felt like a threat.

Most of us don't experience anxiety to such a degree, but it still shapes our lives. Think for a moment of the things we tend not to do. The emails we don't answer, the places we don't go, the positions we don't apply for, and the risks we don't take. We come up with all sorts of excuses like 'I'm tired or too busy', but often we're just scared!

So why do we worry, and what stops us from facing our fears? Here are some of the reasons why I cling to anxiety:

1. I want to avoid disappointment.
2. I'm not sure that God has heard me.
3. My husband/family/friends don't worry enough – so I feel I need to do it on their behalf.
4. I'm worried that life is going badly – something has to go wrong!
5. I think that life is going well. Too well . . . so what have I missed?
6. I'm bored.
7. I feel like everything depends on me.
8. Worrying is a way of taking control (I *want* everything to depend on me).
9. Manageable concerns (like phone bills) distract from bigger ones that I can't fix (such as sadness, loneliness, sickness or death).

Each worry promises to be the last. I tell myself, 'If I can get through *this*, I'll be contented. If I can just pass this exam, then I'll be at peace.' Yet when one fear is resolved, another takes its place. Corrie ten Boom, a Dutch Christian author, argues, 'Worrying doesn't empty tomorrow of its sorrow, it empties today of its strength.'[5]

> *I worry about everything and anything. It could be, what am I going to do tomorrow? But also, will I be able to finish my course? . . . Will I even be OK enough tomorrow to get up and get stuff done? If I don't get anything done, what will my family think? What if I fail my course? What if I am never going to be strong enough to manage life? What if I can't be there for people?*

We might blame money problems, social media or even terrorism for our fears, and these things can play a part. But there's a far deeper source . . .

Anxiety in the garden

Ever since Adam and Eve rebelled against God, fear has been a part of our lives. In fact, it's the first emotion described in the Bible:

> Then the man and his wife heard the sound of the LORD God as he was walking in the garden in the cool of the day, and they hid from the LORD God among the trees of the garden. But the LORD God called to the man, 'Where are you?'
> He answered, 'I heard you in the garden, and *I was afraid* because I was naked; so I hid.'
> (Genesis 3:8–10, italics mine)

When we stop trusting our Father, we become orphans instead of his children, and the world becomes a scary place. Suddenly Dad seems like a stranger. Instead of running to him, we run from him, but we're too small to care for ourselves. Dazzled by independence, we toddle straight into the traffic, and our worries bear down on us like trucks. We try to dodge them, but they keep coming. Without help from outside, we'll be crushed by their weight.

The right kind of fear

This is fear at its worst. But there's a kind of fear that's also – well, good! Some things *should* fill us with awe – most of all, God. The Bible talks about 'fearing God' more than 300 times and says that it's 'the beginning of wisdom' (Proverbs 9:10). This 'fear' isn't about being horrified or wanting to run away. It's about responding to God's glory and goodness with humility and respect.

Godly fear puts our other worries into perspective, because the Father promises to protect us, and he is greater than any evil force. He invites us to bring our fears to him (1 Peter 5:7) and promises to deal with them (Philippians 4:19). Yet while we might 'know' this in our heads, we listen to other voices instead. Think of how the devil tempted Adam and Eve. He asked, 'Can you really trust your Father? What if he lets you down? Wouldn't you be better off looking after yourself?' The devil's tactics haven't changed, and he still uses fear as his chief weapon (Hebrews 2:14–15). If we listen to him, then these fears will take hold of us too.

Thinking it through

What am I most afraid of?
What do my worries reveal about the things I value most?

Which relationships and situations do I avoid
  because of fear?
What would it look like to give my fears to God?
  How would this change the way I see my
  world?
How does fear of the Lord help me to put other
  worries into perspective?

Fear at the extreme: anxiety disorders
Thirty-five years ago anxiety wasn't recognized
as a disorder. Now, along with depression, it's
officially the most common form of mental illness
(*DSM*).[6]

Who?
• Anxiety and depression have increased by 13%
  since 1993.
• Up to a third of the population will suffer from
  an anxiety disorder at some time.[7]
• Rates are increasing: 37% of British people report
  feeling more frightened than they used to.[8]

What?
Anxiety is the body's natural response to danger and
it helps to protect us from physical harm. However,
if it continues over a long period, it can have a negative
impact on almost every area of life.
  There are six major types of anxiety disorder:

Generalised anxiety disorder (GAD): Long-lasting
anxiety that's not anchored to one particular issue or
situation.

Obsessive-compulsive disorder (OCD): Intrusive thoughts ('obsessions') that drive sufferers to perform certain behaviours ('compulsions').

Panic disorder (anxiety attacks): Repeated episodes of intense panic or fear, which normally happen suddenly and without warning.

Phobia: An exaggerated fear of an object, activity or situation that really presents little or no danger. This is the largest category of anxiety disorders (affecting between 5% and 12% of the population worldwide).

Post-traumatic stress disorder (PTSD): An extreme anxiety disorder that occurs after a traumatic or life-threatening event. Symptoms include flashbacks or nightmares.

Social anxiety disorder (SAD): Fear of being viewed negatively by others and humiliated in public, also known as 'social phobia'. Performance anxiety (better known as stage fright) is the most common kind.

Summary

God protects us, and he made us to have a healthy humility or 'fear' of him. When we lose sight of him, we're dominated by worldly fears and we try to deal with them alone.

Now we turn to our third impulse: control.

Control

In the section on hunger we saw that restricting food can give us a false sense of control. This desire for control works out in other behaviours, which can include obsessive-compulsive disorder (OCD).

As a teenager, I suffered from severe OCD. I couldn't use public toilets, or touch door handles or anything else that might be covered in 'germs'. If I did, then I thought that something terrible would happen to me or to the people I loved. To stay safe I developed complex cleaning rituals, like scrubbing my hands and body in a particular order. This process took hours – and every 'mistake' meant starting afresh. I knew it was irrational, but I was scared to ask for help. After all, if I couldn't understand myself, what would others think?

I've been able to break my compulsions – thankfully. However, I'm still scared of losing control and I still employ little 'habits' to make me feel secure. I often deal with big fears (sickness, relationships, life choices) by transferring them to smaller and more manageable categories (like home or personal improvements). Here's the logic: I can't control when I'm going to die, but I can control my hair colour. I can't stop myself getting older, but I can fight it with serum and supplements. I can't stop my loved ones from getting cancer, but if I follow certain routines, then maybe they'll be safe.

Let's say we're going on holiday. Everything is turned off, but as my husband honks the car horn, I do a 'last-minute check'. I inspect the cats, the oven, the lights, the washing machine, the windows and the doors. But the more I check, the more I need to check again. As we drive away, I'm muttering about the house burning down, but what's really worrying me is something else. It's the difficult conversation I've had with my sister. The bills that we hadn't budgeted for. The friend who's going through a painful divorce. These circumstances are beyond my control, so I look to the things that I *can* manage instead.

Control in the garden
Our culture paints God as the ultimate control freak, but wanting control is actually a *human* problem. The story of Adam and Eve is a prime example. They think that they'll find freedom by breaking God's law. But as they break his rules, they start *making* their own:

> The woman said to the snake, 'We may eat fruit from the trees in the garden, but God did say, "You must not eat fruit from the tree that is in the middle of the garden, *and you must not touch it*, or you will die."'
> (Genesis 3:2–3, italics mine)

God told Eve not to *eat* the fruit; he said nothing about touching it! However, Eve adds to God's law, making it heavier than God had intended. Yet Adam too is at fault. When God gave the original warning in Genesis 2, Adam was there and Eve was not. Adam was meant to take responsibility and protect his wife. Instead, he watches as Eve rebels. Both abuse the control that God gives them. The woman is meant to trust, but instead she grasps; the man is meant to protect, but instead he shirks. And the curse only deepens these patterns: '[God said to Eve] "You will desire to control your husband, but he will rule over you"' (Genesis 3:16, NLT). After the fall the woman wants to dominate, while the man becomes even more selfish. Right from the outset we see that humanity wrestles with control.

The right kind of control

God has ordered every part of our world and he calls us to reflect this in our work and home lives. He commissioned Adam and Eve to rule the world under him (Genesis 1:28), and this remains true, even after they sin (Psalm 8:6–8). Jesus promises that we will rule with him (Revelation 3:21) and he even describes our salvation as 'reigning on thrones' (Matthew 19:28)! However, there's a huge difference between caring for our world under God's lordship and trying to control it in our own strength.

Thinking it through

How does it feel to be 'out of control'?
In what ways have you seen God directing the course
    of your life?
Have you ever wanted to take control from him?
    How and why?
Why is control so appealing? In what ways is it a
    false hope?

Control at the extreme: obsessive-compulsive disorder (OCD)

Who?
Two in 100 adults are affected by OCD, and one in every 100 children and teenagers.[9]

What?
Sufferers have repetitive, intrusive and unwelcome thoughts/impulses that make them anxious and distressed. Examples include fear of contamination,

---

21

anxiety about causing harm, and upsetting, sexual, violent or blasphemous thoughts. To relieve their anxiety, they develop mental or physical rituals ('compulsions'), such as washing, checking, counting or thinking in certain ways.

'Pure O' is when sufferers have distressing thoughts, without appearing to use rituals. However, they often cope by doing these things mentally or by avoiding certain situations.

There is also a form of religious OCD where sufferers are overwhelmed by fear of angering or disappointing God. This may lead them to avoid church or other Christians.

Whatever its expression, OCD can have a devastating impact:

My OCD must have made me quite difficult to work with at times. One colleague called me a 'pain in the neck', which puzzled and upset me at the time (the OCD was undiagnosed then), and she relented, but looking back I can see how I would have been!

I had to tell my line manager when I came off medication and was feeling unwell. Some days I could barely function, and it was starting to affect my performance.

It is one of the few flashpoints in our marriage, and has been responsible for a lot of arguments, and even delaying having a family, as contamination fears were too large for me to relax.

Summary
Since the Garden of Eden humans have wanted to be in charge. We might joke about having 'control issues' but,

in all seriousness, we want to take God's place. When our hearts are exposed, this makes us ashamed.

Shame

I'm standing in the supermarket queue when I hear my name.

'Emma! Emma *Scrivener!*'

It's almost teatime and the aisles are packed. Everyone swivels to see who's speaking.

'*Emma Scrivener!*'

Three aisles away, a man is waving. His face looks vaguely familiar, but I'm not sure why. I wave back and my daughter starts crying. 'Lord,' I pray, 'give me patience.'

'Emma Scrivener! It's *you*, isn't it? I saw you on the TV!'

(I talked about my eating disorder in a programme that had aired a few days earlier.)

'Anorexia! Ever since I saw it, I've been thinking about *your anorexia!*'

A slow burning flush creeps across my neck and cheeks.

'You don't *look* anorexic. But you can't tell, can you? The thing with *anorexia* is . . .'

Seven minutes later and he's still shouting about *your anorexia*.

People are staring at my shopping basket and wondering if potatoes are a sign of recovery or relapse. My daughter is screaming at the top of her lungs. And my prayer has changed from 'Help' to 'Please, Lord, beam me up.'

An encounter in the supermarket – based on information I shared – reduced me to a quivering wreck. But what if my whole life was on display? Every cruel word, every lie, every jealous thought? What if my heart was exposed in all its wickedness?

I'd crawl under a rock and never come out.

This is how it feels to be ashamed. The bits you want to keep hidden are completely exposed – and *everyone sees*:

> Shame is never appropriate in polite company. It's a brand, a stamp, a stain. It makes you want to give up and crawl away and hide and apologize until your speech dries up. It's a lowered gaze, a shuffle, an internal folding. It sets you apart, and you can't go back.[10]

When others see us as we really are, we long to cover up. Yet this hasn't always been the case.

Shame in the garden

In the beginning, 'Adam and his wife were both naked, and they felt no shame' (Genesis 2:25).

Adam and Eve are naked before God, in every sense. He sees their bodies and he sees their hearts; yet he loves them unconditionally. This is paradise, and we yearn for it too. Instead, we hide and wear masks, even with friends. We worry that if they see us as we really are, they'll reject us. But imagine if we could be naked and not feel ashamed.

The TV presenter, Sue Perkins, sums it up:

> The crowning ambition in my life is to be able to be with another person. That's all we all want. We say we want world peace, but in truth we want to be totally exposed in front of someone who says, 'Actually, you're all right.' The creepy intimacy of really knowing someone and them really knowing me . . . I would be incredibly sad if I got to the end of my days and didn't have that.[11]

Adam and Eve have this intimacy with God. However, when they disobey him, everything changes. They realize that they're naked, and they try to cover up . . .

> Then the eyes of both of them were opened, and they realised that they were naked; so they sewed fig leaves together and made coverings for themselves.
> Then the man and his wife heard the sound of the LORD God as he was walking in the garden in the cool of the day, and they hid from the LORD God among the trees of the garden. (Genesis 3:7–8)

Adam and Eve don't just cover their actions, but *themselves*. That's because shame is personal. It's not just what we do; it's who we *are*. When their sin is exposed, they blame one another. They hide behind fig leaves and they hide behind lies:

> But the LORD God called to the man, 'Where are you?'
> He answered, 'I heard you in the garden, and I was afraid because I was naked; so I hid.'
> And he said, 'Who told you that you were naked? Have you eaten from the tree from which I commanded you not to eat?'
> The man said, 'The woman you put here with me – she gave me some fruit from the tree, and I ate it.'
> Then the LORD God said to the woman, 'What is this you have done?'
> The woman said, 'The serpent deceived me, and I ate.' (Genesis 3:9–13)

As I read these verses, I want to shout, 'You idiots! What are you thinking? Just own up!' Surely none of *us* would make the same mistake?

'Not so,' says the Bible. When *our* sin is exposed, we also hide from the light:

> This is the verdict: light has come into the world, but people loved darkness instead of light because their deeds were evil. Everyone who does evil hates the light, and will not come into the light for fear that their deeds will be exposed.
> (John 3:19–20)

When you are exposed, how do you cover your shame? Maybe you hide behind your performance: *I try to do everything absolutely perfectly so that no-one can be ashamed or shame me.*

Maybe you retreat into self-hatred and despair: *I have a habit of feeling like everything is my fault and that I should just hide from everything/everyone so I can't make things worse.*

Maybe you try to destroy the root cause – even if it's another person. Journalist Jon Ronson explains:

> I once interviewed a prison psychiatrist, James Gilligan, who told me that every murderer he treated was harbouring a central secret – which was that they felt humiliated. 'I have yet to see a serious act of violence that was not provoked by the experience of feeling shamed or humiliated, disrespected and ridiculed,' he said. His conclusion: 'All violence is an attempt to replace shame with self-esteem.'[12]

'Now hold on,' you might say, 'I've never tried to kill anyone.' Perhaps not, but there are other ways of lashing out. Imagine you're running late for an appointment, but have lost your keys. How do you react? Maybe, like me, you attack other people. You storm through the bedrooms, firing accusations: 'Who moved my keys? I know where I left them and they're not there! Someone must have taken them.'

Or maybe you criticize yourself: 'What an *idiot*,' I mutter (sometimes even out loud). 'I can't even look after a set of keys! I can't do anything right. I'm a total waste of space.'

Author Dan Allender writes about shame in the context of sexual abuse (which we'll consider in Part 2). He says that shame is so powerful that it can only be covered by an equally violent emotion such as hatred or rage. Allender argues that we'd rather hurt ourselves than acknowledge our shame, and we'd rather attack others than have it publicly exposed.[13]

We all know what it's like to harm ourselves verbally, yet when we harm ourselves physically, it provokes a shocked response. Are the two really so different?

Seeing the cuts on my body just felt 'right'. After all, I was messed up and dirty . . . it was deeply satisfying to make the outside of my body look like how it was inside.

Our natural response to nakedness is to cover our shame, without coming to the grace and cleansing of God. We do this by punishing ourselves (or others). A friend sums it up well:

Punishing ourselves is just another way of justifying ourselves and living without God. Every time I cut, I was trying to save myself.

The 'right' kind of shame

But as with hunger, anxiety and control, not all shame is bad. When we say to one another, 'Have you no shame?' we're using the word in a positive sense. 'Good' shame recognizes that there is both appropriate and inappropriate disclosure. There are parts of us that *do* need to be covered, at least in certain circumstances, or with certain people. However, inappropriate shame causes us to hide even the parts that we should share. It causes us to lash out rather than own up.

Thinking it through

What makes you feel ashamed?

How do you try to 'save yourself' from shame?
   In what ways does this 'work'? In what ways does
   it fail?

'We say we want world peace, but in truth we want
   to be totally exposed in front of someone who
   says, "Actually, you're all right."' Can you identify
   with these words? What stops you from being
   naked before others?

What would it be like to be truly known and truly
   accepted? How would this change the way you
   relate to God, to others and to yourself?

Shame at the extreme: self-harm (SH)

Who?
- 1 in 12 UK adolescents regularly self-harm – the
  highest rate in Europe.
- Most are aged between 11 and 25.[14]

- 50% of young people aged 15–21 know someone who self-harms.
- Girls are four times more likely to self-harm than boys.

What?

Deliberately injuring yourself in order to find relief from difficult or painful emotions.

Includes: cutting, burning, scalding, scratching, biting, scraping, taking dangerous substances, hitting, hair-pulling, head-banging, breaking bones. It might also mean taking unnecessary risks, EDs, alcohol or drug abuse. Cutting is most commonly done in private. Self-poisoning is most commonly treated at hospital emergency departments.

Why?

Before self-harming, sufferers experience emotions that feel 'dangerous' or 'wrong'. Self-harm provides a temporary feeling of release, but then brings more shame – which starts another cycle:

When I am feeling annoyed, or sad, or overwhelmed, or out of control, I cut myself and I get relief. Unfortunately, that relief is extremely short-lived and immediately followed by revulsion, but when things are at their worst, the guilt and disappointment are an acceptable pay-off for the relief.

The first incident may happen by accident, or after seeing others do the same thing. However, to get the same effect, sufferers may need to go further each time.

I remember self-harming from about the age of six onwards . . . My mother was unwell, and I also learned that the way to get attention was to be physically unwell/in pain. I started to self-harm more seriously in my late teens, and this time it was to punish myself or as a cry for help . . . I restarted at the age of about twenty-six or twenty-seven . . . when I was worried about my sexuality or when I was afraid that God would ask me to do something really scary. I'd hurt myself . . . to punish myself before anyone else could.

Self-harm can feel like a familiar and reliable friend. It can also be a form of self-medication (as the body releases endorphins to help deal with injury or stress). Sufferers treat one kind of pain (emotional) with another (physical). But by harming themselves, they never really confront the original hurt.

Once I'd self-harmed, I could worry about that and not what had led me to do it in the first place. The other issues didn't go away; they just got temporarily displaced.

Summary

When we disobey God, our sin is exposed and we're filled with a terrible shame. God offers to cover us, but instead we want to cover ourselves. We'd rather hurt ourselves than receive God's healing, and we'd rather attack others than acknowledge our shame. This brings us to our next struggle: anger.

Anger

I read an article recently about 'the things that scare men'. At the top of the list was 'a woman's anger'.

'Glen,' I said, 'Isn't that ridiculous?'

Silence.

'Glen,' I shouted (just in case he hadn't heard). 'Says here that men are scared of women's anger. Hahahahahahaha. You're not scared of me, are you?'

I was laughing till I saw his face. Then I stopped.

'It's one of my biggest fears,' he said. 'I'll do nearly anything to prevent it.'

At first I was shocked: after all, I don't *choose* anger as a deliberate strategy. Yet later that day I remembered something I'd written:

> Depression can be cold, empty and watery. It renders
> you helpless, immobile and pathetic. *Anger* feels very
> different. It's hot and sticky, concentrated and full.
> It propels you forwards. With anger, you can *do*
> something. It feels good. It is energizing. It gives
> you a target, a scapegoat (even if it's yourself).
> For 'nice' girls in particular, that's seductive, but
> dangerous.[15]

Perhaps, like me, you don't think of yourself as angry. At times we might feel 'frustrated', 'disappointed', 'aggrieved' or 'upset'. But *angry?* Absolutely not!

Jesus says, 'Don't be so sure.' He tells us that *everyone* is full of anger – including Christians:

> You have heard that it was said to the people long ago, 'You
> shall not murder, and anyone who murders will be subject

to judgment.' But I tell you that anyone who is angry with a brother or sister will be subject to judgment. (Matthew 5:21–22)

Perhaps, we blame our anger on people and circumstances: 'pushy' sales assistants, 'overzealous' traffic wardens and 'those idiots' on the motorway. Again, Jesus says, 'No'. Others don't cause our anger – it starts *within* us (Matthew 15:18–20).

Anger in the garden

Think back to Adam and Eve. When they wanted the forbidden fruit, nothing – including God – would stop them. Yet, when their sin was exposed, they immediately lashed out:

'The serpent deceived me!' says Eve.

'This woman you put here!' replies Adam.

Their response tells us two things about anger. It starts when someone blocks our goals (exclusion). However, it deepens when we're shown up in front of others (exposure).

When we're excluded and exposed, we cover ourselves, instead of looking to God for shelter. Our anger acts like armour, concealing the shame underneath. Yet it's not always obvious:

I feel like nearly all of me is beneath the surface. I am a naturally content person, and so was mostly just shocked when I got older and I couldn't keep a grip on the world or on my own sanity any more. I come across as gentle, [but] . . . I am incredibly angry.

Anger is a clenched jaw as well as a clenched fist, a sour attitude as well as bitter words. It leaks out as often as it explodes. Sometimes we turn it on ourselves (e.g. with self-harm). Sometimes we turn it on others (e.g. using sarcasm, verbal aggression or actual violence). In all these cases *someone* has done something wrong – and *someone* has to pay.

The right kind of anger

Anger is a God-given emotion, and all of us have felt it. It can be a normal reaction to difficult situations, and it helps us by alerting us to pain or hurt. We can use it as an excuse for sin, but it isn't always sinful in itself. Look at Ephesians 4:26. This doesn't say, 'Don't be angry.' It says, 'Be angry, but in your anger do not sin.'

When we see injustice or oppression, we're right to feel upset. Righteous anger can lead us to repentance, to right wrongs and to defend the weak. In Psalm 7:11 and Mark 3:5 God himself is described as being angry. But there's a big difference between his anger and ours.

God's anger is directed at those who rebel against him or threaten his beloved children; ours is usually about self-protection and fear. God's anger is a feature of his love; ours is often a feature of our pride. When *God's* righteousness is questioned, his anger is fair, measured and just. When *our* righteousness is questioned, we lash out without limits. God's anger brings restoration and healing. Human anger often causes destruction and further hurt.

Thinking it through

What makes you angry? (Give an example from the past week.)

What do you do with your anger? Do you suppress
it – or vent it? In what ways?
How is our anger different from God's anger
(see also Ezekiel 3:18–21; Romans 12:17–21)?
What does God's anger achieve (see Romans 2:12)?
How does this help us when we're tempted to
lash out?

Anger at the extreme

Who?
- 45% of us regularly lose our temper at work.[16]
- 33% of Britons are not on speaking terms with their
  neighbours.
- More than 80% of drivers have been involved in road
  rage incidents.
- 25% have committed an act of road rage themselves.
- One in eight experience violence at work.[17]
- 53% of employees have been victims of bullying at
  work.
- 7% of the UK workforce (1.3 million) have been
  physically attacked by a member of the public.[18]

Warning signs
- Regular loss of temper, often in similar situations.
- Physical fighting, vandalism or property destruction.
- Harming other living things, such as animals.
- Using violent words or making frequent threats
  towards others.
- Relying on anger to make us feel better.
- Avoiding situations because we're afraid of our
  anger.

- Anger-linked health issues like hypertension or digestive problems. (Chronic anger is linked to heart disease, stroke, depression, self-harm, substance abuse, colds and flu, higher stress levels and negative relationships.)

Types of anger

Passive-aggressive anger: expressing anger indirectly and in a controlled way, for example through sarcasm.

Aggressive anger: letting anger determine behaviour in a way that harms others, such as punching, yelling or throwing objects.

Suppressed anger: choosing to suppress or ignore anger.

Assertive anger: choosing to acknowledge and discuss anger in a healthy way.

Summary

We use our anger to hide sin, but God's anger exposes it. We're angered by wrongdoing, but only God's anger brings justice in its place. When we use our anger to 'set the world to rights', we invariably fail. This brings us to our final struggle: despair.

Despair

Feelings of despair are difficult to describe if you've never had them:

One of the hardest things is not being able to articulate the experience: the effect it has on those closest to me; the feelings of being a burden and causing trouble/ inconvenience to colleagues, etc. The times of sheer blackness which reduce me to a mumbling stupor, or the panic attacks.

It's more than feeling sad or low. It's . . .

clinging on and wanting to let go
feeling useless and lazy and not really ill
hating yourself and hating the world and not
   seeing any way out
being crushed by a weight that gets heavier and
   heavier
falling, with no-one to catch you
needing others, but worrying that you're a burden
being trapped inside your head
pretending to be OK when everything feels wrong.

I once asked a despairing friend, 'What helps?' He replied, 'Nothing. Nothing helps.' That's what makes despair so painful. It *is* helplessness. It's the feeling that engulfs us when nothing we do makes a difference.

Picture a man locked in a room. For hours he pounds furiously on the door. But eventually, instead of trying to escape, he collapses in dejection. He does so because *he's given up hope.* With anger, we're hopeful that our protests will be heard. With despair, we may be committed to our goals, but we've lost hope of reaching them.

Despair in the garden

We see this pattern in Genesis 4:

> Adam made love to his wife Eve, and she became pregnant
> and gave birth to Cain. She said, 'With the help of the
> LORD I have brought forth a man.' Later she gave birth
> to his brother Abel.
>   Now Abel kept flocks, and Cain worked the soil. In
> the course of time Cain brought some of the fruits of the
> soil as an offering to the LORD. But Abel also brought
> an offering – fat portions from some of the firstborn of
> his flock. The LORD looked with favour on Abel and his
> offering, but on Cain and his offering he did not look
> with favour.
> (verses 1–5a)

Does God have a preference for steak over broccoli? Why
does he accept Abel's offering and not Cain's? To understand, let's go back to Genesis 3. When Adam and Eve
disobey God, they try to hide behind fig leaves. But plants
are not enough! The Lord covers them in animal skins,
showing that only blood can deal with our sin. Yet in
Genesis 4 only Abel learns the lesson. Abel's blood sacrifice
(Leviticus 4:35) says, 'I need the Lord to cover my sins.'
Cain's plants show that he'd rather cover himself. God
rejects Cain's offering, and Cain becomes angry. But that's
not all he feels:

> But for Cain and his offering He [God] had no respect
> or regard. So Cain was exceedingly angry and indignant,
> and he looked *sad and depressed*. And the Lord said to
> Cain, 'Why are you angry? And why do you look sad and
> depressed and dejected? If you do well, will you not be

accepted? And if you do not do well, sin crouches at your door; its desire is for you, but you must master it.' (Genesis 4:5–7, AMP, italics mine)

When God refuses to accept Cain on his own terms, Cain kills his brother. Just as he chose his own sacrifice, he chooses to vent his anger rather than confess it to God. When he's punished (verse 12), his rage turns to despair.

We might not have committed murder, but, like Cain, we've had murderous thoughts. We want acceptance on our own terms and, like Cain, we'll do anything to get our own way. When our sin is exposed, we too lash out. Then, when our anger subsides, we're filled with despair.

The right kind of despair
Despair is painful, yet in some situations it's an appropriate reaction. There are some things that I cannot do (like earning my own goodness, controlling my life or fixing the world). I *ought* to despair of these!

Suffering can also provoke the right sort of despair. The Bible gives us many examples, such as Job, a man who lost his health, family and possessions. Job doesn't pretend to be OK, but he does take his despair to God. When he cries out, his 'friends' tell him to cheer up, but the Bible insists that he did not sin. In fact, God criticizes the advice of his friends (Job 42:7).

Acknowledging loss is part of good emotional health, as Jesus shows when he weeps at a friend's death (John 11:35). All of this represents 'good despair'. However, there is a kind of despair that is not God's will for us. This despair turns us inwards instead of towards God. It refuses to receive even gospel comfort.

Thinking it through

Are there hurts in your life that *need* to be grieved? Or areas where you need to despair of your own strength? Ask God to reveal these to you and to help you bring them to him.

Does your faith allow for times of real sadness and grief? Why or why not?

In what ways have you known God's comfort when you've been struggling with despair?

How would you describe the relationship between anger and despair? Where do you see them in your own life?

Isaiah 53:3 says that Jesus was 'despised and rejected by mankind, / a man of suffering, and familiar with pain'. How does this bring us comfort and encourage us to bring our pain to him?

Extreme despair: depression

Please note that depression is a complex issue with a variety of causes, some of which are beyond our control. It may be a form of despair, but it is not always the same thing.

We can despair, without being clinically depressed. And we can have depression, but still know Christian hope.

Who?

- Depression is the most common mental health disorder. It affects nearly a fifth of adults in the UK,[19] one in five older people living in the community and two in five living in care homes.[20]

- Over the past forty-five years, suicide rates have increased by 60% worldwide. In 2010 a US veteran killed himself every sixty-five minutes.[21]
- Every year 5,000 people in the UK take their own lives. Almost a quarter of these are men aged between 16 and 24. Men aged between 20 and 24 are four times more likely to kill themselves than women – even though more women attempt suicide and more suffer from depression.[22]

What?
Depression affects people in different ways. These range from lasting feelings of sadness and hopelessness to losing interest in the things you used to enjoy. At its mildest you may feel persistently low in spirit, while at its most severe you can despair of life itself.

People experience depression differently – for me it is a black, hopeless place with no perspective. It is very difficult to describe. There is a constant state of pain. Simple tasks are impossible. Getting out of bed is a mammoth effort. At its worst, I found breathing in and out all day and not harming myself to be all I could manage. God is completely out of reach. The Bible is no comfort because everything within screams that it is lies. Depression feels like being in the grip of the devil.

It creates a sense of profound isolation – from God, from friends, from those I love and who love me.

Common types of depression

Depressive episode: The formal name given by doctors when they make a diagnosis. It may be described as 'mild', 'moderate' or 'severe'.

Dysthymia: A mild but ongoing type of depression (usually lasting more than two years).

Bipolar disorder ('manic depression'): Sufferers experience severe 'highs' (mania) and 'lows' (depression). Around 1 in 100 is affected.

Psychotic depression: Severe depression accompanied by hallucinations or delusions (psychosis).

Perinatal or postnatal depression: Depression occurring during pregnancy or after the birth of a child. This affects between 10 and 15 out of every 100 mothers.

Seasonal affective disorder: Also known as SAD, this often develops in autumn and winter; it is a reaction to low levels of natural light.

---

* * *

Twilight reflections

Hunger, anxiety, control, shame, anger and despair. We see them first in the Garden of Eden, but they're still with us today, because we are born into Adam and Eve's rebellion against God. What they want, we want, and what they do, we do too. This is what Christians call 'original sin', and it's shorthand for 'we're all messed up'.

Original sin isn't a religious excuse for self-hatred, but a way of expressing our universal struggles. When we admit that we *all* need help, we can face our own issues and care for others. Instead of thinking of ourselves as somehow 'better' or 'worse', we recognize that we're all in the same predicament.

For those who think they're OK, the Bible says, 'Your problems are much deeper than you think!' But for those who fear they are beyond help, it says, 'Your issues are everyone's issues.' This is a huge comfort, especially as we think about mental health. It stops us from dismissing such struggles as unusual or surprising. It also stops us from labelling sufferers as 'especially sinful'. Unfortunately, this can happen, even amongst Christians (who really should know better).

> *The hardest responses to deal with have been those from evangelical Christians whose understanding of depression is that it is a sign of spiritual weakness or an indicator of disobedience or sin. I can't see how such views fit with the many desperate cries to God in Scripture – Elijah, Job, Jonah . . . the Psalms – yet it is these responses [from Christians] that have damaged and hurt me the most.*

Our struggles may vary, and we *will* handle them in different ways. But we're all in the same situation. When it comes to mental health, there is no 'us' and 'them'. There's only 'us'.

> We are *all* hungry – doubting God's promise to
>   provide.

We are *all* anxious – refusing to rest in God's
protection.
We are *all* desperate for control – not wanting God
to rule.
We *all* feel shame – yet reject God's covering.
We *all* get angry – ignoring God's justice.
We *all* despair – refusing to hope in God's future.

True healing comes only when we can admit our own
failings. So allow me to lead the way:

My name's Emma. I'm hungry, anxious, controlling,
ashamed, angry and filled with despair. I'm lost in the
dark, and when I try to fix myself, it only makes me worse.

How about you? Can you admit to the same?

Lost in the dark

What's my problem?
When I know things are wrong in my life, why can't I just
stop?

Why do I keep worrying about things that don't matter?
Why can't I control my temper or become more thankful? Why can't I stop nagging my husband? Why can't I
resist the cravings that harm me and other people?

Paul talks about this in Romans 5 – 8. For four chapters
he explores the Christian's divided nature. Our first birth
is in Adam, but our new birth is in Christ: we sin, but we
are counted righteous; we have flesh, but we also have the
Spirit. At times it sounds as if Paul is describing a double-
headed monster, but really he's describing you and me. He

writes, 'I want to do what is good, but I don't. I don't want to do what is wrong, but I do it anyway . . . Oh, what a miserable person I am!' (Romans 7:19, 24, NLT). This is the desperate state of the Christian. Deep down we want to do right – that's a sure sign of the Spirit's work in us – but sin is a power that is bigger than us. Until we see Jesus face to face, we will feel its effects.

According to our old nature, we are trapped by a power that we can't overcome. But through Christ we have a new way to live. This is another angle on the truth we've already discussed: there are both chains and choices; we are both sick and sinners. If we want to move forward, we have to acknowledge both sides:

> One big struggle once I had been 'diagnosed' was accountability to God for my sin. Where did my illness end and my sin begin? Did having a medical reason absolve me? Did it make it not my fault? 'I'm sorry, Jesus, but you can't accuse me of this one – I'm poorly. I can't help it.' No, of course not! But where does that leave me – sinning over and over, unable to prevent it? Well, yes . . . but not because I was depressed! The truth was (and is) that I am broken . . . even when I am 'well'. I still sin over and over. I can never match 'the law'. I always need Jesus.

Sickness and sin: a case study

Meet Clare and Ruth, two friends who get together for dinner. They decide to try a new seafood restaurant and order the clam chowder (which is dangerously under-cooked). That evening both become unwell, and over the next few days both lose their appetite. Clare recovers with no ill effects. But Ruth finds it hard to start eating again. She drops a dress size and is complimented on her new shape. Losing weight becomes an obsession. When her friends say they're worried, she tells them she's fine. Gradually, she develops a serious eating disorder.

Is Ruth 'to blame' for her struggles? You could say no, and with good reason. It's not her fault she got sick, and there are other factors that made it more likely. Maybe she has allergies or particular digestive complaints. Maybe she's under pressure from work or family. Maybe she lives alone (unlike Clare, who was nursed back to health). Maybe she has been bullied or has experienced abuse. Maybe she lives in a culture that admires a particular sort of body shape.

Ruth is not to blame for her food poisoning or her eating disorder. But neither is she just a simple victim. Even in her sickness she has choices. She can choose to acknowledge that she has a problem or she can choose to deny it. She can choose to settle for life with an eating disorder or she can choose to resist it. She can choose to accept help or she can choose to refuse it. She faces many challenges and cannot recover alone. Yet she has a vital part to play in her own recovery.

Choices and chains

If I trip over a pavement slab and twist my ankle, it's not a sin. Nor is it sin to struggle with body image or hunger or mental health. However, there can be sin in the ways I react to being hurt. I can use my pain as an excuse to behave selfishly or badly. I can say, 'I deserve to feel better, whatever it takes and whomever it harms.' Or I can recognize my wrong responses and take them to God:

The lies I tell to cover up my actions.
The choices I make that strengthen bad patterns.
The self-pity I wrap like a cloak round my heart.

My pride in my own strength.
My fury when others try to help.

In all of our struggles there are choices and chains. If we emphasize one at the expense of the other, we see only half of the picture. Remember what Jesus said in Matthew 15:19: 'For out of the heart come evil thoughts – murder, adultery, sexual immorality, theft, false testimony, slander.' Our hearts are sick and we can't fix them. When we try, it's like performing keyhole surgery . . . on ourselves!

If we say that 'sin' is simply making bad choices, we overestimate our ability to rescue ourselves. That's when we invent strategies to cope.

However, if we think of ourselves as purely 'sick', we underestimate our role in our own mistakes. That's when we write sick notes instead. Allow me to explain . . .

Sick notes: permission to stop

At school I hated team sports. Every week I came up with new reasons to be excused: 'Emma can't play netball because she has a tropical disease. Emma coughed up her kidneys at breakfast and will have to miss tennis.'

Happily, netball is no longer part of my routine. But I face other demands, like loving my husband, managing my finances and organizing my time. At points these challenges seem overwhelming. When they do, I write myself sick notes, not from exercise, but from life.

Here are a few:

'I'm afraid I can't do X because . . . I'm too tired . . . I'm busy . . . it's a bad time . . .'
'I'd love to help out, but I'm just not that sort of person . . .'

> *'We can't get involved because that's not how we do things round here . . .'*
> *'I would, but . . . it's just not what I'm used to.'*

Sometimes my sick notes are deliberate (avoiding a difficult conversation by not answering the phone). But sometimes they're unconscious. Anorexia *can* be an example. I didn't pick it like I'd pick out a scarf, yet it worked as a sick note, written across my body. It pressed 'stop': on growing up and expectation and uncertainty and fear. It said, 'Emma can't do these things. She needs to be excused.'

Of course, it's not just those with eating disorders who write sick notes. Think of the excuses that Adam and Eve offer to God:

> 'How am I supposed to do my job, with the woman you put here?'
> 'We wouldn't be in this mess if it wasn't for that serpent.'

Adam and Eve could have owned up and asked for forgiveness. Instead, they hid behind excuses and false weakness. We often do the same thing. Let's say I'm the youngest child in my family: the 'baby'. For years I've resented the assumption that I'm incompetent. Yet even when I leave home, it's a stamp I can't quite shake off. In the workplace and with friends I look to others to tell me what to do. I say I hate being treated like a baby . . . but in some ways it 'works' for me too.

Sick notes aren't just for people with small ambitions, but also for those who aim too high. If I look like I'm strong, people may make demands I can't meet. However, if I say that I'm weak, I can protect myself from challenge and from expectation.

The actor Jeff Bridges puts it well:

You're attracted to something, but at the same time right along with that comes that feeling of, 'yes, but are you going to be able to pull it off?' You keep it in the dream line, it's kind of safe; but (if you succeed) . . . where are you gonna go from there?[23]

When my anorexia was at its worst, I was studying full-time, working as a children's minister and determined to prove my own worth. I was scared of missing the mark *and* I was scared of surpassing it. Anorexia was a way of excelling in one area (weight loss), and a sick note from everything else. This is the sick note's appeal. It gives us permission to stop *and* it protects us from our own success.

Sick notes are one way of responding to struggles. They concentrate *just* on our chains. But what if we take the opposite approach? What if we focus purely on our *choices*? That's when we look to strategies instead.

Strategies: pretending to be strong

If the sick note says, 'I can't – so you must do it', the strategy says, 'I can cope – all by myself!'

Hungry? I'll supply my own needs.
Anxious? I'll protect myself.
Out of control? I'll take charge.
Ashamed? I'll pay for my own sins.
Angry? I'll deliver justice.
Despairing? I'll make my own future.

Whether subtle or obvious, strategies can be very seductive, especially if we're 'religious'.

For me the church that I attend still encourages perfectionism –
doing the best Bible studies, praying good prayers, attending
all the meetings and managing a quiet time each day. Some
days I only manage to yell, 'Help me, Lord.'

Strategies might seem perfect, but they're not. They're built on self-reliance and the *appearance* of strength. They won't allow us to say, 'Help me, Lord' or to ask for support. I say 'they', but I'm really talking about me!

My body was mine and mine alone. It made me powerful and untouchable. The more I shrank it, the stronger I became . . . Other people might die from anorexia, or sink without trace. *I* was different . . . I didn't need help. No-one would force it upon me. No-one would tell me how to live.[24]

Eating disorders can be strategies, but there are many others too. These include workaholism, perfectionism, being 'nice' or relying on our wits or our appearance to navigate life.

Having it both ways

We might think of sick notes and strategies as alternatives. But they're often paired. Initially, I pursued thinness as a *strategy*: a way of feeling strong, powerful and in control. Yet over time it became a refuge from my compulsions – a *sick note* from life. At one stage my 'recovery' was a way of proving how strong I was (through resolutions and sheer grit). When this failed, I went back to anorexia as a sick note. Back and forth I swung, between sick note and strategy, strategy and sick note.

Experiences like mine should make us question what Christian change actually looks like. At points I appeared to be full of Christian resolve (but it was really a strategy). At other times I looked like I was 'letting go and letting God' (when in fact I was writing myself a sick note). Of course, there is true recovery and there are true expressions of Christian strength and weakness. Nevertheless, sometimes our new behaviours are ways of handling life without Jesus or without his cross. Before we resolve simply to 'turn over a new leaf', we need to go deeper. We also need to ask 'why?' and 'how?' What's driving this change and how does it happen?

Next steps

Our problems plunge us into darkness, but our solutions are just as bleak. So how do we move forward? How do we make good choices and break old chains? That's what we'll now explore. But be warned: midnight comes before the dawn, and, in the same way, we go deeper into the darkness before we reach the light. So, as we travel towards resurrection hope, we come to the cross.

2 Midnight
A Saviour who enters the darkness

When I share my story, it provokes different responses. Some whisper, 'It's a relief to hear that you can be a Christian and still have problems. I thought it was just me.' Others want something more. One woman stopped me halfway through my testimony. 'I don't get it,' she said. 'What do you mean, you *met* Jesus?'

I'd been talking about a time when Jesus became real and personal to me. I used the phrase 'I met him', and, understandably, she wanted to know what I meant.

'Great question,' I said. And it was. But I didn't know how to put my answer into words. My fear was that I'd give the wrong impression – as though Jesus had flicked a switch and all my troubles disappeared. I said, 'Well, I met him . . . in the Bible. And then I was different. I mean, I still struggled afterwards. But I *met* him, you know?'

She didn't. So I tried again.

'Jesus didn't wave a magic wand and zap me from a

cloud. He *joined* me in my mess. That's where he works – in broken people. And he's a broken Saviour.'

I flashed my most winning smile and prepared to move on. 'Does that answer your question?'

'No,' she smiled back. 'It doesn't.'

I wish I'd given her a better answer. But here's some of what I'd like to have said . . .

Our sin separates us from God, which means that there's a huge gap between us. So, how do we get across? Other religions answer by claiming to be ladders. They say that we can climb to God by using good works as rungs. Christianity says the opposite: we can't do anything to close the gap, and no amount of climbing will help. If we want to know God, then he must come down to us.

At the cross Jesus does exactly this. Instead of whisking our problems away, he becomes a man, a human being, and meets us in our mess. As we look at his suffering, we're entering the bleakest point of history – and the darkest chapter of this book. But keep going, because there's light ahead. In fact, we can only reach this light by going *through* the darkness.

Hunger

It's hard to think of Jesus as needy or hungry. After all, he's God's Son! But remember what we learned about hunger in chapter 1? It reveals our dependence and points us to God. This is exactly how the Son relates to his Father: 'The Son can do nothing by himself; he can do only what he sees his Father doing' (John 5:19). The Father–Son language here gets us to the heart of God's nature. Jesus has always been the Spirit-filled Son, receiving his life from his Father. This unbreakable union of three Persons – the Father, Son and Holy Spirit – is called the Trinity. It's a way of saying that God is a Family of love – a tri-unity. It means that God's life has always been a life of mutual dependence.[1]

We might see dependence as weakness, but from before the world began Jesus has relied on his Father. This is the pattern of his earthly ministry too. Like us, he's born as a tiny baby, vulnerable and naked. Like us, he experiences hunger and thirst. He starts his public ministry by fasting (Matthew 4:1–11), and ends it by gasping for water on the cross (John 19:28). The devil tempts him by appealing to his hungers, just as he does with Adam and Eve. Yet Jesus has a very different response: 'Jesus answered, "It is written: 'Man shall not live on bread alone, but on every word that comes from the mouth of God'"' (Matthew 4:4).

In the garden Adam and Eve try to feed themselves (remember?); but in the wilderness Jesus takes his hungers to God. He trusts his Father with all of his needs, even when it costs him his life. Instead of feeding himself, he is torn apart like bread. He does this so that hungry sinners can be filled (John 6:51, 53–55).

When Jesus rises from the dead, he cooks a meal for his disciples and eats with them. It's a wonderful picture of reconciliation and celebration, and it points to the time when our hungers will be fully met:

They will never again be hungry or thirsty;
    they will never be scorched by the heat of the sun.
For the Lamb on the throne
    will be their Shepherd.

He will lead them to springs of life-giving water.
And God will wipe every tear from their eyes.
(Revelation 7:16–17, NLT)

Thinking it through

What are you hungry for? How do you try to satisfy
your hungers?
How does it help us to know that Jesus understands
our hungers?
Where does Jesus look to be filled? What does this
teach us about who he is? What does it teach us
about ourselves?
Read Psalm 23. Imagine Jesus praying it as he walks
through the valley of darkness and looks ahead to
the feast. What enables him to keep going?
Take time to bring your hungers before him now.
Pray.

Anxiety

Think of the most stressful situation you can imagine. I
don't mean moving house or facing deadlines (although
these are taxing enough!). Picture a condemned man,
sitting alone on death row and counting down the minutes
until his own death.

This is what Jesus faces – and worse. Instead of a lethal
injection, he'll be humiliated and tortured. And as well as
physical death, he'll experience spiritual death: separation
from his beloved Father. In fact, the night before
he is crucified, he is so distressed that he sweats blood
(Luke 22:44).

Then Jesus went with his disciples to a place called
Gethsemane, and he said to them, 'Sit here while I go
over there and pray.' He took Peter and the two sons of
Zebedee along with him, and he began to be sorrowful and
troubled. Then he said to them, 'My soul is overwhelmed
with sorrow to the point of death. Stay here and keep
watch with me.'
(Matthew 26:36–38)

No-one has ever been more vulnerable than God's Son. In
this situation who could blame him for shutting down or
running away? Yet instead, he faces his fears and prays
about them. Three times he says, 'My Father, if it is
possible, may this cup be taken from me. Yet not as I will,
but as you will' (verse 39).

Our reaction to anxiety is to protect ourselves. Jesus
does the opposite. He lays his fears before his Father.
Then he willingly endures hell to bring us his peace.

When Jesus rises from the dead, he pursues the disciples
who betrayed him. What would we expect him to say?

'Why did you let me down?'

'Wait till my Dad catches up with you?'

'I'll never trust you again?'

To the friends who betrayed him, Jesus says, 'Peace'
(John 20:19), and he says 'Peace' to us too (Colossians
3:15).

Thinking it through

How does Jesus handle anxiety? What can we learn
from his prayers and his example?
On the night before he dies Jesus gives his followers
this promise: 'Peace I leave with you; my peace I

give you. I do not give to you as the world gives.
Do not let your hearts be troubled and do not be
afraid' (John 14:27). What makes his peace so
different from the peace of the world?
Read Psalm 34 and picture Jesus as the Lord who
encamps around us to protect us. At the cross
he suffers so that we are kept safe. Spend time
reflecting on this and thanking him now.
Pray.

Control

Imagine you are Lord over all creation. With a touch you
can heal the sick. With a word you can still the storm.
Heaven and earth hang upon your every command. How
would it feel to have this much power? Wouldn't you want
to hang on to it? Wouldn't you guard it with your life?

Jesus does exactly the opposite. He gives up control.
He *rejoices* to do his Father's will, even though it costs him
his life.

When I'm wrongly accused, I long to justify myself and
take control. But consider Jesus, passed from court to
court, soldier to soldier and cell to execution. On the
cross he was stripped of his power and unable even to
draw breath. His enemies believed they were in charge;
his friends feared that events had spiralled out of hand.
He was pinned before a baying mob, yet he offered no
defence.

No matter how powerless we might feel, we have
never been this weak. It looked like God had been out-
manoeuvred and evil had won. However, Peter tells us
the truth:

Jesus of Nazareth . . . was handed over to you by God's deliberate plan and foreknowledge; and you, with the help of wicked men, put him to death by nailing him to the cross. But God raised him from the dead, freeing him from the agony of death, because it was impossible for death to keep its hold on him.
(Acts 2:22–24)

Christ's death is the ultimate surrender. He appears weak, but in submitting to his Father, he triumphs. He is raised up as the world's true Ruler (Acts 2:36; Philippians 2:9–11) because he follows his Father's will, and all of creation is under his loving control. We can trust him to reign over our world and our hearts.

Thinking it through

How do you feel about the word 'submission'?

Jesus yields complete control to his Father. Does this change your view of submission? In what way?

Jesus says, 'If you try to hang on to your life, you will lose it. But if you give up your life for my sake, you will save it' (Matthew 16:25, NLT). In what ways do you try to hang on to your life (by keeping control)? What does Jesus promise if we submit control to him?

Read Psalm 46, thinking of the Lord Jesus standing firm in the midst of the chaos. Commit to him the things that you try to manage alone.

Pray.

Shame

The last book of the Bible describes Jesus, enthroned in heaven and worshipped by all creation. His eyes are like 'flames of fire', his voice thunders 'like mighty ocean waves', and his face is 'like the sun in all its brilliance' (Revelation 1:13–16, NLT). All who see him worship him, saying,

> Worthy is the Lamb, who was slain,
>   to receive power and wealth and wisdom and strength
> and honour and glory and praise!
> (Revelation 5:12)

It's a dazzling depiction. Yet this same Lord is shamed in a way that we can barely imagine.

Soldiers stripped him naked and gambled for his garments. They put a scarlet robe on him, twisted together a crown of thorns, set it on his head and beat it into his skull. They spat on him, placed a staff in his right hand, knelt in front of him and jeered, 'Hail, king of the Jews!' Then they crucified him with criminals and left him to die.

Crucifixion is a terrible picture of degradation and humiliation. Yet, in Jesus' hands, it becomes something else. Instead of being crushed by shame, Jesus *scorns* it: 'Because of the joy awaiting him, he endured the cross, disregarding its shame. Now he is seated in the place of honour beside God's throne' (Hebrews 12:2, NLT).

Christ's mission required humiliation and death, but his scars have become his glory. Through the cross he scorns shame on our behalf, and makes *us* like *him*: 'God made him who had no sin to be sin for us, so that in him we might become the righteousness of God' (2 Corinthians 5:21).

Thinking it through

Read Mark 15:1–40. In what ways is Jesus shamed? How
  does he overturn shame and bring about its defeat?
What are you ashamed of? What stops you from
  bringing these things to God?
Psalm 32 tells us that our sins were counted against
  Jesus, so that we could know his unfailing love. Read
  this psalm and bring your sin and your shame to him.
Pray.

Anger

When *I've* been wronged, I rush to defend myself. Jesus,
by contrast, stayed silent:

> He was oppressed and afflicted,
>   yet he did not open his mouth;
> he was led like a lamb to the slaughter,
>   and as a sheep before its shearers is silent,
>   so he did not open his mouth.
> (Isaiah 53:7)

When *I'm* angry, I pour hatred on my enemies. Jesus cries,
'Father, forgive' (Luke 23:34).

When *I'm* offended, I lash out. Jesus tells his followers
to put away their swords (John 18:11).

When *I'm* accused, I hit back. Jesus remains calm: 'When
they hurled their insults at him, he did not retaliate;
when he suffered, he made no threats' (1 Peter 2:23).

What makes Jesus so different from us? How can he
forgive even his *murderers*? We're told in the second part

of this same verse: 'Instead, he entrusted himself to him who judges justly.'

When I'm angry, I trust in myself. I proclaim my innocence, even when it's false. Jesus is perfect, yet he endures God's righteous anger for our sin. He is wrongly accused, imprisoned and executed, but he trusts in his *Father* to put things right.

As sinners, we deserve to be judged. Yet Jesus takes his Father's righteous anger in our place. Whatever we may hold against others, it's nothing compared to what we've been forgiven. So, when we're tempted to judge *ourselves*, we remember that Christ has paid for our sins. When we're tempted to judge *others*, we look to the cross and 'leave room for *God's* wrath' (Romans 12:19).

Thinking it through

How does Jesus respond to injustice? How does this
   help us when we have been wronged?
How do you feel about handing judgment over 'to him
   who judges justly'? What is stopping you from
   doing this?
Read Psalm 73, knowing that Jesus is our Judge, our
   Sacrifice and our Strength. What frustrations can
   you lay before him now?
Pray.

Despair

How can Jesus be described as despairing? If he's God, then can't he see that everything will be OK?

Jesus trusts his Father completely, but this doesn't exempt him from sorrow. The very reverse! He enters suffering *because* he is God. No-one but Jesus can bear the weight of our sin, and no-one but Jesus would choose to.

As sinners, we know some of the pain of our separation from God. But we can't begin to imagine what this means for Jesus. For the first time in all eternity he is severed from his Father's love. He's always been perfect, yet he *becomes* sin. By taking our place, he endures the despair of hell itself.

We saw earlier that on the night before he dies Jesus says that his soul is 'overwhelmed with sorrow to the point of death' (Matthew 26:38). On the cross he cries out, 'My God, my God, why have you forsaken me?' These words are taken from the Psalms: the hymnbook of the Old Testament. In them God's people pray out their pain. They speak of darkness, drowning, desperation and grief:

> I am worn out from my groaning.
> All night long I flood my bed with weeping
> and drench my couch with tears.
> My eyes grow weak with sorrow;
> they fail because of all my foes.
> (Psalm 6:6–7)

Astonishingly, God's Son picks up these prayers and makes them his own. *He* bears our tears, our sin and our despair. But he doesn't turn in on himself. He looks to a future that he can't yet see. He cries out to his Father, and he dies to bring us hope.

When John describes the resurrection of Jesus, he tells us *when* it happened: 'early on the first day of the week, *while it was still dark*' (John 20:1, italics mine). Jesus comforts Mary when it is still dark, and it's often in the darkness that he comforts us too. Even when we feel downcast and despairing, he reassures us of his hope: 'He has delivered us from such a deadly peril, and he will deliver us again. On him we have set our hope that he will continue to deliver us' (2 Corinthians 1:10).

Thinking it through

How does Jesus respond to suffering?
How does his suffering speak into our despair?
Read Psalm 22, knowing that Jesus is the One who is praying. Bring your tears to him now, knowing that he carries them and grieves with you.
Pray.

Light in the dark

Can't You Sleep, Little Bear? is a story that my daughter loves. It's about a little bear who's scared of the dark:

'Why are you scared, Little Bear?' asked Big Bear.
'I don't like the dark,' said Little Bear.
'What dark?' said Big Bear.
'The dark all around us,' said Little Bear.[2]

Little Bear's fear makes him look for repeated reassurance from Big Bear. Finally, Big Bear shows Little Bear the enormous moon. Little Bear realizes that even when there is darkness in his room, there is still light outside.

When we're struggling, we can feel like Little Bear. The dark is all around us, and we want someone bigger to switch on the lights.

We're going to get personal now. So let me ask, have the lights been switched on for *you*? Do you know the light of Jesus even *in* your darkness?

I ask this, because I knew lots *about* Jesus before I really knew *him*. Similarly, we can understand the facts of the gospel, but miss the wonder of Jesus Christ dying *for us*.

Knowing Jesus is not about experiencing warm fuzzy feelings. There have been many points when I've felt far from God, yet have trusted that he was holding onto me. It's a bit like being married: whether loved-up or arguing, our wedding vows hold. In the same way, I know that Jesus is committed to me, whatever happens and no matter how I feel. How about you? Can you say the same? Is Jesus Lord of *your* life?

If you don't yet know Jesus and you want to, then drop everything – including this book. Ask him to show himself to you and be your Lord. Here's a sample prayer:

Dear Jesus,
I know that I am a sinner and I need your forgiveness. I believe that you died for my sins and rose to give me life. I want to turn from these sins and live for you. Please would you be my Lord and my Saviour?
Amen.

Now tell another Christian. The Bible says, 'Faith comes from hearing . . . the word about Christ' (Romans 10:17), so start by reading one of the Gospels and get along to a Jesus-centred church. Many churches run seeker courses for those with questions, such as 'Christianity Explored' or 'Alpha', and these are a good way of meeting other Christians. But whatever happens, don't settle for anything less than a living relationship with Jesus. Nothing is more important.

Thinking it through

If you already know Jesus or have just prayed this prayer, then spend some time praising him.

Starting to see the light

We've travelled through the darkest hour of the night – well done for staying with me! However, the real work happens as we bring our hearts before God.

Facing our mess isn't easy, but Jesus has joined us in the darkness. At the cross,

He takes our hunger and offers us his fullness.
He enters our anxiety and gives us his peace.
He obeys his Father and frees us to live for him.
He is cursed, to take away our shame.
He takes God's judgment so we can be forgiven.
He carries our despair and gives us real hope.

As morning breaks, we can begin to live in this hope. It's now time to think about the day ahead . . .

3 The early hours
A Saviour who shines

The night before my wedding I couldn't sleep. For months we'd been planning, and finally the big day was almost there. In those early hours I paced the floor, wondering how my life would change. I thought about the family I was leaving behind and the one I was starting. I took stock of where I'd come from and where I wanted to be. I said goodbye to my old self and started to embrace my new identity.

As we wait for the dawn, let's take stock. The day we're entering isn't just a rerun of our past; it's a new day, and as we're joined to Jesus, we're new too. Let's look at four new challenges we'll face as Christians – and four new 'gifts' that help us to deal with them.

Four challenges

Challenge one: we expect change
When Kate Middleton married Prince William, the service was broadcast worldwide. As the couple exchanged vows,

Kate's life was transformed. She took on William's name and gained all that was his: his wealth, his power and his kingdom. In an instant an ordinary girl became a princess. No wonder we were transfixed!

When we are united to Jesus, the same thing happens. We get all that he has, and he takes all that belongs to us. On the day I married Glen (as penniless students), there was a slightly different dynamic. I gave him my debts . . . and he gave me his. But with Jesus it's different. He takes our debts and, in return, he gives us his perfect life. Whatever our history, it's as if we've never done anything wrong. Amazing!

Never lied or raged or despaired or hungered.
Never lashed out at the people we love.
Never said things that are too terrible to speak.
Never ignored God or tried to take his place.

By trusting in Jesus, we become part of his family. His Dad becomes our Dad, and the Father sees us as he sees his own perfect Son. This might seem shocking, especially if we've felt or done things that feel too dark to be covered. However, through Christ's death, they already are covered. This very moment we can come to him and say, 'Here. Take my mistakes. Take my shame. Take my sin and my sickness. Take my mess.' And he does.

Jesus loves us even in our sin, but he also calls us to leave our old lives behind. Again, think of what happens when we marry. We don't act as we did when we were single; instead, we commit to one person for the rest of our lives. In the same way, becoming a Christian involves new commitments and change on every level. This takes us to our second challenge.

Challenge two: we expect mess

I've compared us to Kate Middleton on her wedding day. But we're far from spotless brides. In fact, the Bible says that God's people are more like prostitutes (see Ezekiel 16 and Hosea 1)! This sounds harsh, but it's a picture of the ways we've been unfaithful to God. Time and time again we run from him and into the arms of other lovers. We're tempted to act like the people we used to be and not the people we have become.

Put yourself in the shoes of the new bride who's just married her prince. She is 100% princess, but will she always *feel* like one?

No.

Likewise, does she instantly *act* like a princess?

No. It takes time to feel like royalty and it takes time to act like royalty too.

When we exchange vows before God, we are changed. However, marriage is about more than just one day; it's a lifetime of becoming new. When I was dating my husband, I wore emotional (and physical) make-up. But when we were married, he saw me as I really was. This was terrifying for us both!

It's hard to change old habits and it's hard to step into a new identity. It's hard to be naked in front of someone else. We can only do it because our partner is committed to us – for better or for worse, for richer or poorer, in sickness and in health. If we're worried that we will be abandoned, we won't trust our spouse. But if we know we are loved permanently and unconditionally, then we can take off our masks. This leads to challenge three.

Challenge three: we expect weakness

In the wedding vows the couple share themselves, knowing that neither is perfect and both will make mistakes. It's the same for us. As we share our hearts, we expect brokenness and mess, but Jesus rescues us *in* our frailty:

> Brothers and sisters, think of what you were when you were called. Not many of you were wise by human standards; not many were influential; not many were of noble birth. But God chose the foolish things of the world to shame the wise; God chose the weak things of the world to shame the strong. (1 Corinthians 1:26–27)

Jesus doesn't ask us to be strong or self-reliant, and we shouldn't ask this of one another. If we do, the consequences can be devastating:

> *I remember a friend, when I first told him my story, just holding me and crying with me. He was willing to hold some of my pain as my brother, and that gave me courage to stand. Conversely, I also remember being told that if I was a real Christian, I could pray and not feel like this. Suffice to say I actually tried suicide the day after – I felt like I'd let everyone down, including God.*

'Real' Christians follow a Lord who was crucified 'in weakness' (2 Corinthians 13:4) and comes for the helpless and lost. They don't despise frailty or struggle; in fact, they expect it.

Challenge four: we expect suffering

In romantic novels marriage often looks easy. But remember those vows:

For better, *for worse.*
For richer, *for poorer.*
In *sickness* and in health.

Before Glen and I married, an older couple warned us to expect pain as well as good times, and this helped us to persevere. If we'd expected instant bliss, we'd have given up at the first hurdle or assumed that something was terribly wrong. Yet as Christians, we can do exactly this. We panic when times are hard and wonder if God really wants us. He does – and suffering is an unavoidable part of following him.

Listen to what Jesus tells his followers: 'Whoever wants to be my disciple must deny themselves and take up their cross and follow me' (Mark 8:34).

As Christians, we are joined to Jesus, so we go where he goes. This might sound daunting, but he equips us with four incredible gifts.

Four gifts

A new Father: God

On my wedding day Glen's parents gave me a hug and welcomed me into their family. When we're united to Jesus, the Son of God brings us to his Father, making him 'our Father' too. We've touched on this truth already, but how does it actually make you feel?

Mostly, [I think of God as] a wonderful, lovely, kind, forgiving, perfect Father . . . but sometimes he's a bit scary and annoyed at me.

I grew up with an image of God as all about rules. I am now beginning to understand love and grace, but I still battle with this image.

If your earthly dad has hurt you or let you down, your response may be mixed. This is understandable, but your heavenly Dad is very different. To see what the Father is like, we look at the Son (John 14:6, 9). All that we have learned about Jesus – his love and beauty, his power and mercy, his sacrifice and glory – are true also of his Father. So, if you think of the Father as being harsh or 'all about rules', think again. He is love, and he pours this love out upon his Son and upon us.

We catch a glimpse of this love in John 17, when Jesus prays to the 'Father . . . [who] loved me before the creation of the world' (verse 24). It's a privileged peek into the family of God, but we're not left outside. In the very same verse Jesus asks his Father if we can join in: '[Father], I want those you have given me to be with me where I am.'

And the Father says, 'Yes!' 'See what great love the Father has lavished on us, that we should be called children of God! And that is what we are!' (1 John 3:1).

Each time I look at my daughter, my heart lifts. I love her unconditionally – whether she's crying or sleeping, giggling or screaming. She's too small to speak, and she can't pay me back for feeding or washing her. But she doesn't need to! All she can do is receive. In the same way, we come to our heavenly Father, exactly as we are. We don't need to make an appointment. We don't need to use special words or clean ourselves up. He makes his home with us (John 14:22–24) and provides all that we need (John 16:23–24). He is strong enough to shield us

(John 10:28–30). He is tender enough to comfort us. He looks at us and is filled with love. When we call God *Abba*, we're reminded that we're *his*.

A new Brother: Jesus

When I was younger, I dreamed of having an elder brother who would stick up for me and fight my corner. Someone who would speak for me when I had no voice and put himself in danger, just to keep me safe. Jesus is like this brother.

Traditionally, the elder brother plays the peacemaker or 'mediator' in family disputes. Jesus makes peace for us on the cross (Hebrews 2:11), and he prays for us, without ceasing:

> Even now my witness is in heaven;
>   my advocate is on high.
> My intercessor is my friend . . .
>   he pleads with God
>   as one pleads for a friend.
> (Job 16:19–21)

> Christ Jesus . . . is also interceding for us.
> (Romans 8:34)

> [Jesus] is able to save completely those who come to God through him, because he always lives to intercede for them.
> (Hebrews 7:25)

When prayer feels impossible, our Brother prays for us. When we're far from God, he carries us into his arms. When we sin, his wounds buy us forgiveness. When we feel lost and forgotten, he owns us proudly before heaven.

A new Helper: the Holy Spirit

God the Father shelters us, and God the Son speaks for us. But that's not all! God the Spirit is given to all believers (John 14:16), and he helps us. When we're filled with fear, the Spirit brings us peace (John 14:27). When we're hurting and choked up, he puts words to our pain (Romans 8:26). He tells us who we are (John 14:6) and makes us more like Jesus (2 Corinthians 3:18). He shows us how to talk to God (Galatians 4:6), and he corrects us when we go wrong (John 16:8).

American author and preacher Tim Keller puts it like this:

> Many people say that the Holy Spirit gives us power, and that's true, but how does he do that? Does he merely zap us with higher energy levels? No – by calling him the *other* Advocate [or Helper], Jesus has given us the great clue to understanding how the empowering of the Holy Spirit works. The first Advocate [Jesus] is speaking to God for you, but the second Advocate [the Holy Spirit] is speaking to *you* for you.[1]

We hear many verdicts on our lives, but these are usually negative or critical. The Spirit speaks to us gently and with love. Paul sometimes describes the Christian life as a battle between the old me (the 'flesh') and the Spirit of Jesus (who now lives in me). The old me says, 'You're an orphan and must look after yourself.' The Spirit says, 'You're God's beloved child and he will care for you.'

A new family: the church

So we have God the Father, the Son and the Holy Spirit. Our fourth gift is often criticized or misunderstood, so we'll spend a little longer on it. Let's think about church.

Christians are united to Jesus in a marriage-like relationship. But when we are joined to him, we are also joined to other believers. We're part of a clan of brothers and sisters that stretches across the world and across time. This means that when we read about Christians in the Bible, they're not strangers, but relatives. And, unlike some relatives, they can't be avoided!

When Jesus came to earth, he went to the local synagogue, even when they tried to kill him. He didn't hold out for 'the perfect church'. Instead, he committed himself to a very *im*perfect church, one that he died for. There will always be areas of church that can be improved, and it's important to talk these through. But there's a difference between running something down from the outside and strengthening it from within. Church is where everyone belongs. It's not flawless, but neither are we.

How do you feel about *your* church? Is it a warm family gathering? Or a place that fills you with panic, where you need to perform or pretend?

I don't know how to be in church when I'm struggling.

I don't want to be on the edge . . . but I struggle to interact socially. I look longingly at others chattering away, laughing and hugging as I sit alone in the pew pretending to read the notices!

It's hard to be around others, especially when we feel broken or vulnerable. Sometimes they remind us of things that we want but don't have: a partner or a family, a secure home or a job. At these times our hearts might say, 'Stay away – church will make you feel worse.' Instead, we experience God's love and grace in community. The single person starts to pray for the couple who are struggling in their marriage. The childless are reminded that a new baby is a blessing, but not a saviour. Life is still hard, but our trials are tempered with a new patience and realism. We carry one another instead of battling alone:

> My church saved me: they took me to the doctors and stood with me on the path to recovery. For the first month of being in hospital I received a letter daily from one of my fellow interns. These letters showed me love and community like I never knew before . . . my non-Christian family cannot comprehend why people who are not related to me would go out of their way to give me a home, money and relationships.

When you're not at church, a vital part is missing. Even if you're completely unlike the others in your fellowship, you fill a place that no-one else can. We're *meant* to be a ridiculous, rag-tag mixture: that's what sets us apart!

> God has placed the parts in the body, every one of them, just as he wanted them to be . . . The eye cannot say to the hand, 'I don't need you!' And the head cannot say to the feet, 'I don't need you!' On the contrary, those parts of the body that seem to be weaker are indispensable, and the parts that we think are less honourable we treat with special honour . . . Now you are the body of Christ, and each one of you is a part of it.
> (1 Corinthians 12:18, 21–23, 27)

However long we've been away and whatever our background, church is where we belong. We're committed to walking alongside one another, and this, not warm, fuzzy feelings, is what makes it home. If, like me, you find community daunting, then why not pray about it? Make a list of the things you love about your church and thank God for each one.

Here are thirty reasons why I go to church; I'm sure you can add many more!

1. To remember the past.
2. To let go of the past.
3. Because I can't love God until I know that he loves me.
4. To be connected.
5. To quiet my soul.
6. To wake me up from self-absorption.
7. To know who I am and where I belong.
8. Because the Bible tells us it's vital (Hebrews 10:24–25).
9. To reflect on my week and see it through God's eyes.
10. To gain hope and strength for what is ahead and for what has been.
11. To learn how to live.
12. To learn how to die.
13. Because the church is less when I'm not there.
14. Because I need my family around me.
15. Because others' words to my soul are more powerful than my own.
16. Because we are united in Jesus.
17. So that I can share my burdens and carry those of others.
18. To see what God is doing in other people.
19. To be challenged.
20. Because the Christian life is not meant to be lived alone.
21. Because my gifts are for the church and not me.
22. Because I need reminding that God is big and powerful.

23. Because I need reminding that God became small and weak.
24. Because we're not all the same and I forget that.
25. Because we're not so different and I forget that too.
26. Because I have a lot of questions and a lot of mess.
27. For the singing and the stories.
28. As a witness to the world.
29. Because everyone belongs.
30. Because church refocuses me and helps me to see life as it really is.

Don't give up on your church: it's where God works.

Summary
When we are joined to Jesus we can expect mess, weakness and suffering. However, we're also equipped with four astonishing gifts:

a Father who loves us
a Brother who prays for us
a Spirit who helps us
and a church that carries us.

These are huge truths, and they'll take time to sink in. But how do we apply them to our daily lives?

How does Jesus sustain me when I face difficulties at work? How does the Father give me strength to care for my elderly parents? What difference does church make if I'm single but long to be married? How does the Spirit help me when I'm filled with anger, shame and despair?

Let's bring these important questions (and ourselves) into the light.

Part 2

LIFE IN THE LIGHT

4 Dawn
Stepping into the light

A day in the life of a child of Adam

I wake up and a thousand needs wash over me like a wave: my alarm's blaring and it's all too much. I roll over and hit 'snooze' . . .

Twenty minutes later:

I'm still groggy, and now I'm in danger of missing my bus. Yet again I sat up into the small hours, watching reruns of a film I'd already seen. Why can't I get to bed at a decent time and get up like everyone else? Other people have got their lives and diaries under control. I'm lazy and hungry and late – but there's no time for breakfast, not if I'm going to make the bus.

I race downstairs and search for my keys. I thought I'd left them on the table, but they're definitely not there. After rummaging through my handbag, I finally find them. Frustrated, I try to slam the front gate, but it won't shut – another simple chore I haven't done. I give it a kick and look up to see my neighbour waving from across the road. At church they've been telling us to reach out to our neighbours, but there's no time, and anyway I'm in a foul mood. More guilt to add to the list! I'm a terrible Christian and human being. I'd be better off staying in bed.

A day in the life of a child of God

I wake up and a thousand needs wash over me like a wave: my alarm's blaring and it's all too much.

I roll over and send up a prayer flare:

'Lord, I don't know how to cope with today: Please help!' I look at the Bible by my bed and it winks back at me. Reading seems like too much right now, but I pull out one of my favourite verses: 'Underneath are God's everlasting arms' (Deuteronomy 33:27). It's enough to get me moving, and I stagger into the shower. *Thank you, Lord, for hot water.* After coffee and cereal, I open the Bible again. It's a passage we've been studying in home group, and it reminds me that I'm not alone. 'Lord Jesus,' I pray, 'Help me to do today in your strength. Amen.' Time to get moving.

It takes a while to find my keys, but I've got ten minutes until my bus arrives and the sun is shining. As I struggle with the front gate, my neighbour waves. Embarrassed, I explain, 'DIY: really not my thing!' She laughs: 'Me neither. John's good with house stuff – if you're free later, I'll ask him to take a look.' I agree, but only if she promises to join me for a cuppa. It's an answer to prayer and it even felt natural!

My appointment is in half an hour and I'm still nervous, but the day is starting to feel less heavy. I remind myself again of God's promises and text a friend to ask if she'll pray for me. As the bus pulls up, I pray for her too. *Thank you, Lord, for giving me the strength I don't have.*

In both situations my circumstances are the same, but my responses are different. In the first one I'm thinking like a child of Adam. In the second I'm letting the Bible tell me who I really am. In the first I'm clothed in my old self, with her old habits and thinking. In the second I'm clothed in my new identity as God's beloved child.

New clothes

When morning breaks, it's time to get dressed. After all, pyjamas are fine at midnight, but not in the afternoon. In the same way, we must live differently now that it's light:

> Do this, understanding the present time: the hour has already come for you to wake up from your slumber, because our salvation is nearer now than when we first believed. The night is nearly over; the day is almost here. So let us put aside the deeds of darkness and put on the armour of light. Let us behave decently, as in the daytime, not in carousing and drunkenness, not in sexual immorality and debauchery, not in dissension and jealousy. Rather, clothe yourselves with the Lord Jesus Christ, and do not think about how to gratify the desires of the flesh. (Romans 13:11–14)

As Christians, the apostle Paul tells us to 'put on Jesus'. This means taking on his identity – stepping out of our old selves (in Adam) and into the people we were made to be (in him). It's great advice, except for one problem. Our old selves may be filthy, but they are very comfortable too. Like smelly trainers, they feel like they *fit*.

I hate buying new shoes, but sometimes I just have to. My old ones let in the rain and they damage my feet. The new ones feel heavy and awkward, and I have to 'break them in' before they feel like 'me'. But I persevere because I need them and because they take me to places I can't otherwise reach. This can be a bit like 'putting on Jesus'. At first it's uncomfortable because he calls us to leave old habits behind and travel to places we don't normally go. But we keep going because we want to move forwards and step into the good life he has for us.

In Ephesians 6:15 Paul says, 'For shoes, put on the peace that comes from the Good News so that you will be fully prepared' (NLT). That's what we'll be doing in the rest of this book. We'll look at how the gospel reshapes our thinking (mind), our self-image (body) and our hearts (emotions). And we'll think about some other helps, including professionals, medication and church community. So shoes on and let's start walking . . .

Putting on new thoughts (mind)
Growing up, I laughed at my granny for talking to herself. But it looks like the joke is on me! In the Bible, self-talk isn't a sign of madness; it's the path to sanity. That's because there's a strong connection between what we think and who we are: 'As a man thinketh in his heart, so is he' (Proverbs 23:7, KJV).

Let's imagine I see myself as 'boring' and 'ugly'. When I meet new people, I assume that they feel the same. So I try to protect myself: I fold my arms, avoid eye contact, mumble and cover up. This makes *them* uncomfortable, so, in response, they withdraw. What's happened is this:

my fears have become reality, because my thinking has changed my actions.

As we saw earlier, since Adam and Eve rebelled, every part of us is broken. It's easy to see this in our bodies (especially as we get older). It's more difficult to spot it in our thinking. Here are some examples:

Seeing things in black and white: e.g. 'I am either "fat" or "thin", "in control" or "out of control", "good" or "bad".'

Focusing on the negative: e.g. 'I may have passed my exams, but I didn't get full marks. I'm a failure.'

Emotional reasoning: e.g. 'I feel bad, so I must be a bad person.'

Jumping to conclusions: e.g. 'A friend didn't return my call. I've obviously done something to offend her.'

Worst-case scenario: e.g. 'If I ask for help, everyone will assume I'm incompetent.'

Overgeneralizing: e.g. 'I've made mistakes in the past, so I'll never be able to change.'

Mind-reading: e.g. 'I'm sure everyone is laughing at my ideas. They must think I'm an idiot.'

Over time these thoughts become part of our mental wardrobe, like smelly trainers that we won't throw away. They're comfortable, so we keep putting them on, and they become automatic, for example, 'I've always been unlucky' or 'You can't teach an old dog new tricks.' However, while they might be true of our old selves, they're not true any longer. In Jesus we're made new . . . and you really can teach a new dog new tricks!

So what do we do when our thoughts run away with us? Here's an example. Imagine I'm shopping with my daughter and she dashes towards the road. Should I simply watch, or follow her obediently into the traffic? No! I go after her. I grab her and I hug her to me and I teach her how to stay safe. Similarly, when my thoughts run into traffic, I go after them. I take *each thought* captive (2 Corinthians 10:5) and I teach them gospel truth.

Perhaps I'm at a party and I don't know anyone there. I can't help feeling awkward, but I can choose how I respond. I can panic and leave, or I can remind myself of the truth: *This is hard – but that's OK. God will help me. I'll give it at least twenty minutes and introduce myself to someone new.* Even with long-term struggles (like wanting a partner) my instinctive thoughts don't need to have the last word. I *can* retreat into self-hatred or self-pity: *There must be something wrong with me and I'll always feel alone.* Or I can acknowledge my hurt *and* speak hope to my soul: *I'm finding this tough, but God hears my prayers and he is with me. I don't know what the future holds, but right now, this is where he wants me.*

The twentieth-century preacher Martyn Lloyd-Jones describes it like this:

> I say that we must talk to ourselves instead of allowing 'ourselves' to talk to us . . . Have you realized that most of your unhappiness in life is due to the fact that you are listening to yourself instead of talking to yourself . . . The essence of this matter is to understand that this self of ours, this other man within us, has got to be handled. Do not listen to him. [On the contrary,] turn on him; speak to him; condemn him; upbraid him; exhort him; encourage him; remind him of what you know, instead of listening placidly to him and allowing him to drag you down and depress you.[1]

Clothed in Jesus, we can challenge old patterns, knowing that we're made new in him. It's not easy, but the alternative is to remain unhappy and stuck. A friend uses the analogy of swimming against the tide:

> As I swam with the flow of anorexia, it was easy and I was good at it, but when I stopped and turned direction, the current became fierce and I faced the hardest battle I have ever faced.

For most of our lives we 'go with the flow', but in Christ we can change direction. We do this by swimming *against* old lies and replacing them with gospel truths. The old me says I'm useless, unacceptable, worthless, purposeless, unstable and vulnerable. But the Bible says I'm useful (Ephesians 2:10), accepted (Romans 5:8), valuable (1 Peter 2:9), purposeful (Psalm 138:8), stable (Proverbs 31:25), hopeful (Hebrews 6:19) and safe (Deuteronomy 33:27). The more I challenge my old thoughts with the gospel, the easier it becomes to swim – until finally, my new identity feels like second nature.

If you're still listening to your own self, then why not write it a letter, challenging its lies? Here's how I addressed my anorexia:

> *Dear Anorexia,*
> *For far too many years I've listened to your nonsense. So take a seat and shut up – because this time I'm doing the talking.*
> *I'm not surprised you're looking shifty. Easy to whisper this sort of nonsense and then slip out, isn't it? 'You're useless. You're ugly. You take up too much room. You're out of control. You're "fat"'. Well, let's see if your arguments hold up, shall we?*
> *First, the 'fat' issue. Don't make me laugh. When I was dying of malnutrition, you said the same thing.*

*'Fat' gets a bad press, but you know what? It's actually
a good thing. Not just in a 'nice-to-fill-out-my-jeans' way, but
the often-overlooked 'you'll-die-without-it' sense. 'Fat' is not a
malignant force, any more than food is the enemy. It's part of
being human and bodily – no more and no less. So you can stop
shaking that stick at me, because I'm not scared any more.*

*What's that? Yes, I am bigger. My old clothes don't fit, and
yes, it takes some getting used to. But you're talking like that's
a bad thing. Actually it's great. Health and fullness and
normality. Bring it on.*

*Tell me this: if I were 'fat', would that be such a terrible
thing? Would the world collapse? Does the sun stop rising
and setting because my jeans are too tight? Is that what you're
threatening me with – dress size? Really?*

*'Fat' is not a feeling. You know it and I know it too. This
was never about body mass, was it? It's about being scared and
wanting control and trying to be strong and to make life work.*

*I don't know how to make life work. But you don't either,
and you're not my boss.*

*Anorexia, my friend, you've been replaced. Instead of a
substitute god who takes all I have and still wants more, the
real God has given everything to make me his. He's far more
beautiful than you. And he won't let me go. But that's precisely
what I'm doing with you.*

Emma

Thinking it through

Here are some questions to ask yourself when you're
tempted to slip into old 'shoes':

Am I confusing a thought with a fact?
How could I see this issue from a different
   perspective? What does the Bible say about it?

What concrete evidence is there to support my
  view?
What do my Christian friends and leaders think?
What are the benefits of thinking this way? What
  are the drawbacks?
Will this still matter in a week, a year or ten years'
  time?
*I am loved unconditionally by the Father and utterly
  secure.* What difference does this make to how
  I feel now?

What does all of this mean for our bodies and emotions?

Loving your skin (body)

Few of us are completely happy with our bodies, and the
world is full of conflicting advice. Magazines tell us that
we're 'perfect as we are', but then suggest that we can be
more perfect if we'd only lose a few pounds/whiten our
teeth/meditate/detox . . . (see their sponsors for more
details). It's exhausting. So how does the Bible help?

Psalm 139 describes our bodies as 'wonderful', and tells
us that they're a big part of how we serve God today
(1 Corinthians 6:20). But the Bible says that our bodies
have a great future too. Perhaps you rub your creaking
knees and think, what's the point? Isn't my body headed
for the ground? No! Listen to this statement of gospel
faith:

At the last day, such as are found alive shall not die, but
be changed: and all the dead shall be raised up *with the
selfsame bodies*, and none other (although with different
qualities), which shall be united again to their souls,
forever.[2]

When we die, our bodies won't be thrown away or replaced; they'll be redeemed and made new. Just as Jesus took on a body like ours, in the future we'll have a perfect body like his (1 Corinthians 15:35–58). In the meantime, we're told to look after our bodies because they belong *to him*:

> Or do you not know that your bodies are temples of the Holy Spirit, who is in you, whom you have received from God? You are not your own; you were bought at a price. Therefore honour God with your bodies.
> (1 Corinthians 6:19–20)

Maybe, like me, you want to glorify God in your body, but find it a struggle. How can we move forward? Is it a case of just 'loving the skin we're in'?

Well, let's try it. Picture your kidneys. Yes, your kidneys (shaped like commas, under your ribs). Talk to them now. Tell your kidneys, 'I love you. I really love you.' Spend time on each one individually, so that neither feels left out. Then multiply those warm feelings by ten. Really, really *love* those kidneys. After you've finished, you can move on to your liver. Next try your bladder, your lungs, your tonsils and your toes. Feel the love coursing through your body!

How was that? I'm guessing you felt silly, but not much different. Choosing to love our bodies is like chasing the wind; it takes a lot of effort, but there's little pay-off. What's more, 'self-care' can quickly become self-punishment instead. 'I'll love my body . . . but only when it's bigger/leaner/fitter/more attractive. I'll love my body . . . if I can only change my nose/my lips/my thighs/my wrinkles/my teeth.'

The world tells us to 'love ourselves', but only if we follow its rules. Every day the advice changes. When I was born, Mum was advised to lie me on my tummy and to drink Guinness (though not necessarily at the same time). When I had Ruby, I was told to stay away from alcohol (and peanuts and shellfish and soft cheese) and lay her on her back. When Mum was growing up, she was told to eat butter, cheese, meat and potatoes. Now we're told to cut out wheat, dairy, carbohydrates, meat, sugar, salt and gluten. Whatever era we live in, 'thou shalt not' cannot make us whole.

The apostle Paul wrote about this 2,000 years ago. He was describing the 'religious' people of his culture . . . but he could equally be describing ours today:

> You have died with Christ, and he has set you free from the spiritual powers of this world. So why do you keep on following the rules of the world, such as 'Don't handle! Don't taste! Don't touch!'? Such rules are mere human teachings about things that deteriorate as we use them. (Colossians 2:20–22, NLT)

When following a new 'body regime', I feel wise and even spiritual. But Paul says these things are self-focused and a waste of time: a truth borne out by my experience. Looking at my struggles with anorexia, I realize that I was most obsessed with food when I was eating least. I spent hours poring over cookbooks, watching baking programmes and thinking about meals, yet refusing to handle, taste or touch. I treated my body 'harshly', but instead of satisfying my hungers, it inflamed them. In fact, it nearly cost me my life.

Over time, I'm learning to value my body, but it doesn't feel easy. As part of this process I wrote it another letter. Perhaps you could try the same thing:

Dear Body,

I'm sorry I've hated you for such a long time.

I'm sorry I tried to starve out your strength.

I'm sorry for saying you were ugly when you were beautiful. I'm sorry for making you my god – and giving you my shame.

I'm sorry for the ways I put you down. 'Baggy brain, empty womb, crumbling bones'. For saying you were weak when you were so strong. For saying you were strong when you were so weak.

I hated you and I harmed you – then I cursed when you gave way. The 'useless' legs that ran and leapt and the 'ugly' arms that stretched and hugged. The 'wonky' teeth and 'rebellious' hair –'I wish it would fall out!'

Clumps on my pillow. 'How I wish it would grow back.'

I'm sorry I took you for granted. I'm sorry I blamed you for what was never your fault.

Thank you for sticking with me when you could have given up. Through anorexia and depression. Through sickness and through sin. Through singleness and through marriage. In the car crash and the hospital ward. When I punched you – and when I painted you. When I stuffed you and when I starved you. When I tried to kill you – and when I begged you not to die.

Dear Body, you're not weak or fat or useless or ugly. You are beautiful and wonderfully made.

I thank God for you. And I pray he will teach me to care for you, as I should.

Thinking it through

Picture your body as a child in your care. Like all infants, it requires regular food, sleep, exercise and love. What would you say to it? How would you look after it?

*I'd go back to when I was thirteen and I'd tell myself that
I don't have to grow up right now, I don't have to go at
someone else's pace, that I can just take my time and I'll
get there. I'd say that I am a marvel because of the character
and the unique personality that God made in me and because
of the body that he made to be beautiful. I'd tell myself to
pray and pray and pray in everything, and I won't regret it.
I'd tell myself that no matter how men treat me, I can always
trust God. I'd tell myself not to be afraid of my body, and
that all the changes in it would one day be things I'd grow
to love, but that I didn't have to let that happen until I
was ready. I'd tell myself not to rush or to let anyone else
rush me.*

If God has made our bodies in his image, then how can we
say that they're 'ugly' or 'useless'? Let's ask him to help us
value them as he does and thank him for all the things they
can do.

Exposing our hearts (emotions)

Having thought about our bodies, we turn now to our
emotions. The philosopher Plato compares these to run-
away stallions. He says that our desires drag us along like
horses drawing carts. There's just one complication: they
pull in different directions! So how can we stop them from
tearing us apart?

Plato taught that our minds should rule our hearts (or
at least try to do so). The world claims the opposite: that
we should follow our hearts, wherever they go. The ancient
approach advises us to *suppress* our feelings; the modern
one tells us to *express* them without limits. The Bible says
that neither is right. Our hearts are too precious to
squash, but too broken to follow blindly.

I was reminded of this recently. I'd spoken at an event and was worrying about what people thought of me. Hungry for reassurance, instead of picking up my Bible, I decided to go shopping. I bought two jars of wrinkle cream and a dress that didn't fit. Why? Because my heart said, 'If you have these items, you'll be someone acceptable. Someone who is strong and confident and beautiful and fun. Angelina Jolie, not Emma Scrivener.'

Have you ever bought into the same lies?

'I feel like another four cocktails will make me more
     interesting.'
'I feel like I need my sister's car/shoes/job.'
'I feel like if I just got married/divorced, life would
     be so much better.'
'I feel like if I was better looking, I'd finally be happy.'

'Follow your heart,' says the world. But here's how the Bible describes those same hearts:

Failed, faint, hard, stirred, sorrowful, lifted, hot, astonished, trembling, melted, rejoicing, offended, bowed, troubled, tender, proud, soft, panting, contrite, sore, overwhelmed, pained, wounded, heavy, sick, despairing, moved, stout, deceitful, stony, bitter, exalted, good, burning, troubled, pricked, anguished and poured out . . .

If you met someone like this, would you trust them with something precious? Hopefully not (unless you own shares in wrinkle cream).

In fact, the Bible goes further still. It says that our hearts are deceptive. When we follow them blindly, they lead us astray:

The heart is deceitful above all things
and beyond cure.
Who can understand it?
(Jeremiah 17:9)

If we follow our hearts, they'll lead us into trouble. However, if we suppress them, we'll run into other problems:

I have always experienced emotions as noise in my head. I shut the negative out and push them aside until they get so loud that the only way to turn them off is to cut.

If we shut out negative feelings, we lose touch with our positive feelings too. Instead of feeling less sad, we feel less of everything . . . less joyful, less compassionate, less hopeful and less alive. Handling our emotions in this way is like pushing down a lid on a pot of boiling water. Eventually it'll overflow (and we'll be burned!).

I pretend the negative feelings are not there . . . then eventually they build up so much that I can't hold them in any more and break down.

The Bible steers us through these extremes. Instead of following our feelings blindly (expression), or pushing our feelings down (suppression), it advises us to listen to them and then talk back. When we do this, it's like lifting a lid off the pot and safely letting out the steam.

Thinking it through

Do you ever squash your feelings? Why is this an appealing strategy? How does it make them worse?

What are your greatest hopes and your deepest fears?
What do they reveal about your inmost desires?
What would it mean for you to acknowledge your
longings, but also speak to them with gospel truth?
Do you allow others to do this? If not, what needs
to change? Pray about this now.

Summary

In this chapter we've thought about taking off our old selves and putting on the new self (or 'stepping into the light'). Now that morning is here, let's actually do this! Beginning with hunger, we'll revisit our old struggles, showing how Jesus changes the way we think, feel and act.

5 Morning
New power for old struggles

We've travelled through the night, and at times it's felt very dark. But throughout it all we've been moving towards one goal: morning and the promise of a new day. As the sun rises, it's time to put into practice what we've been learning.

In this chapter we'll revisit our old struggles with hunger, anxiety, control, shame, anger and despair. This time, however, we're dressed in our gospel armour. We'll bring old lies into the light, but now we'll speak to them with gospel truth. We'll also challenge old thoughts and behaviours, because in Christ we are made new. In all this we'll dare to face the things that scare us most, because Jesus has driven out the darkness and we are children of the light.

The day starts with breakfast, so let's think about how we bring our hungers under Christ's lordship.

Handling our hungers

They're not always what we think
When my daughter was born, she had to learn how to eat. She'd try sucking her fingers and the buttons on her dad's shirt, but what she needed was milk – and only Mum could supply it.

Like Ruby, we sometimes suck on buttons when we need proper food. We look to the world to satisfy us, but only God can meet our deepest needs. Think back to the Israelites in the wilderness . . .

The manna discipleship programme
When God's people, the Israelites, were wandering in the desert, they cried out to him for food. He supplied them with heavenly bread called 'manna', but in their hunger, they panicked. Some tried to store up too much, and some gathered too little. But whatever they did, he gave them just what they required.

Although we can't always see it, God does the same with us today. I think I need a holiday from deadlines. God says, 'No, but I will help you meet them.' I think I need more sleep, or a house with more space. God says, 'No, but I'll look after your family.' I think I need a haircut, better test results or a change of scene. God says, 'No, you just need *me*.'

When Jesus tells us to pray for 'daily bread', he's reminding us that we're a wilderness people and as dependent upon him as the Israelites in the desert (Matthew 6:11). Like them, we are filled with hungers, and like them, we're told to bring our needs to God. However, just as the 'manna discipleship programme' lasted for an entire generation, learning the lessons of 'daily bread' is the work of a lifetime. God's sustenance is ongoing, not just a one-off meal.

Wrestling with our wants

Hungers are another way of talking about emotions. They're the insatiable desires of our restless hearts, and none of us handles them as we should. However, writer Lizzie Jank gives us some great advice. She speaks about teaching little girls to manage their emotions, but her words apply to hungry adults too:

> Little girls need help sorting out their emotions – not so that they can wallow in them, but so they can learn to control them . . . We tell our girls that their feelings are like horses – beautiful, spirited horses. But they are the riders. We tell them that God gave them this horse when they were born, and they will ride it their whole life . . .
>
> When our emotions act up, it is like the horse trying to jump the fence and run down into a yucky place full of spiders to get lost in the dark. A good rider knows what to do when the horse tries to bolt – you pull on the reins! Turn the horse's head! Get back on the path![1]

When our hungers threaten to take us off the path, we must talk to them and steer them back. We don't crush them, but we don't allow them to lead us either. Instead, a bigger and healthier appetite must take their place.

The idea of replacing unhealthy desires with healthy ones is familiar; what's less clear is how we actually do it. When I was dying of anorexia, my counsellor suggested that I make two lists. In the first, I had to write down what my eating disorder took from me. In the second, I had to write down what it gave me. The aim was to show how the disadvantages of an eating disorder outweigh the positives.

The first list read, 'Without anorexia I can . . . go for a curry; see more friends; make my loved ones happier; look healthier and have more energy.' The second list said, 'Anorexia tells me who I am; makes my life safe; overshadows other worries; gives me a sense of power and control; stops me from having to grow up; it's the one area where I'm a success.'

My first list was full of good things, but in comparison to the second, they seemed insignificant. That's because it takes more than the promise of better skin to defy an addiction. If we want to change our hungers, we need to set them on someone more beautiful. Instead of settling for buttons, we need to seek milk.

In Revelation 2 Jesus speaks to a church that has lost its love for him, by settling for other things. Jesus tells them that they can rediscover their true and original love by repenting and doing the things they 'did at the first'. This is also true for us. If we've lost our passion for Jesus, he says to us: *Remember when you first came to me: your joy and enthusiasm, your hunger to know more, the way you pored over your Bible and shared your faith? Do these things again and you'll fall back in love!*

So, as we break our evening fast, this is how we manage our hungers. We take them to God, day by day. We talk back to them and remind ourselves that Jesus will meet our needs. We fix our eyes upon him, and as he feeds us, our other desires start to find their rightful place.

Thinking it through

What hungers are you aware of in your own life?

If my daughter wants food and I give her a dummy, she'll suck it briefly – and then cry again. What 'dummies' do we use as substitutes for God?

When we're physically hungry, how does this change the way we think, act and feel? When we miss time with God and other Christians, how are we affected?

Read Matthew 14:15–21, Exodus 16:13–18 and Philippians 4:19. What do these verses tell us about God's generosity and provision?

Eating disorders

Dear Emma,

I have a question. I don't know if you can be anorexic and then bulimic as well, but that's what's happening with me. Sometimes I don't eat, and then I can't stop, and I feel guilty and I try to exercise it off. I really want to change, but I don't know where to start. Have you got any advice?

Carina*

(*Not her real name.)

Dear Carina,

Well done for tackling your eating disorder: that's a great first step. I'm afraid there's no method of getting better which doesn't involve you feeling a bit rotten (at least at the start). However, just as we learn to think in unhealthy ways about our identity and food, we can learn to think in healthy ways too.

LIFE IN THE LIGHT

The first thing to do is to tell someone you trust. Give them permission to ask you how you're doing, and to help you move forward. Ask them to go with you to see a GP. Book a double appointment so you have space to talk, and if you're not sure what to say, then print out a list of ED symptoms from the Internet and tick the ones that apply to you. Ask what help is available (e.g. dietician/counselling), and see if there are any support groups in your area.

If you're binge eating and/or purging, keep a diary of when, why and where it happens. Share this with a friend, and be specific about how it makes you feel and any triggers there may be. Don't skip meals, and do carry snacks to keep your blood sugars stable. Eat with others when you can, and ask for company/support after meals, especially if you feel panicked.

Plan activities that aren't based around food, and don't go food shopping when you're overtired or hungry; instead, make a grocery list in advance or order food online. It's also useful to plan and prepare meals in advance. (A dietician will help with this if it feels overwhelming.)

If you purge, practise delaying until you can resist it entirely. Start with five minutes, then ten, then twenty, and so on. It takes time and practice, but remember that feeling uncomfortable is not the same as being unable to cope. Break big goals down into smaller ones, for example by limiting your binges to one place and time, or cutting down on how often you purge. Stay calm and remind yourself of the truth. Instead of saying, 'I'm starving and I need to binge', pray and tell yourself the truth: 'I want to overeat – but that's OK. If I don't give in, nothing terrible will happen. The desire will get weaker, and in time it'll go away.'

Keep a record of every little victory, and learn from your mistakes. What was it that made you want to binge and/or purge? What could you change next time? Ask yourself: what do these habits stop me from doing? What would life look like without them? I found it useful to print out Bible verses that talk about identity in Jesus and post them in prominent places (mirrors, fridge, my purse). John 1:12, 1 Peter 2:9, Romans 8:35–39, Ephesians 1:4 and Hebrews 13:5 are favourites!

Recovery is a process, so if you stumble, don't beat yourself up and don't give up. Admit that you're struggling, ask for help and start again. Think of a toddler learning to walk. His parents don't shout at him when he falls – they pick him up and encourage him onwards.

Most of all, keep going. A friend of mine has battled with bulimia for many years, and in her darkest moments she despaired even of life. But step by step she's been rebuilding. And today she says this:

I've experienced/am experiencing true healing: physically, emotionally, spiritually . . . And I am so encouraged in knowing that I'm still a work in progress, and he's not done with me yet.

You're not on your own, and with the help of others, you can do this.
Love,
Emma

Summary

Only God's love can satisfy our hunger and drive out our desires for other things. Just as we need regular meals, we keep going back to him, and he fills us.

A prayer for the hungry

Dear God,
As I start this new day, I'm tired of being ruled by scales and calories. I'm tired of being ruled by food. I'm tired of trying to manage my hungers by myself. I'm tired of starving and stuffing and striving. I'm tired of hiding. I'm tired of lying. I'm tired of trying to save myself and I'm tired of trying to run my own life.

I'm sorry, Lord. Please forgive me for the ways that I have sinned against you and against others and against my own body. Thank you that these things are now in the past. Please change my heart.

Help me to love the body that you have given me.

Help me to see myself as you do.

Help me to challenge old lies and to walk in freedom.

Help me when I'm tempted to turn away from your truth.

Thank you for loving me. Thank you for being with me. Thank you for forgiving me. Thank you for a new day and a new start. Thank you for giving me people who can support me. Help me to be open with them and with you.

Amen.

Next we'll tackle anxiety. Let's see how Jesus teaches us to face the day ahead without giving in to fear.

Answering our anxieties

A TV presenter shows her guests how much junk food they consume in a year. Confronted by vast mountains of sugar and salt, participants are visibly stunned. 'It's just not possible,' they gasp. 'How can we have eaten so much?'

It's an effective tactic. But a year's worth of anything is overwhelming, and worry is just the same. Imagine a table laden not with food, but with cares. Your desperation, your distress and your pain all piled up in one place. No-one can deal with all of this. But sometimes we try. At these times we tend to fall into one of two categories: we become either wall builders or walkovers (pushovers).

Walls and walkovers

When we build walls, we say 'no' to everything and keep others at arm's length (e.g. by hiding behind sarcasm). When we become walkovers, we say 'yes' to everything and then burn ourselves out (e.g. through being 'nice' or 'helpful'). Both extremes are unhealthy, and neither deals with our stress. If we say 'no' to everything, we become isolated and more frightened. If we always say 'yes', we become resentful and worn out. So how can we learn to set healthy boundaries and manage our fears?

1. We recognize that stress is an unavoidable part of life
When life feels messy, I order my socks and my cupboards. I polish and I hoover; I sort and I fold. To my mind, an ordered home is a calm home. But my daughter loves to make mess. So I've been forced to embrace stains and spots – but in the process I've learned something surprising. As I face my anxieties instead of running from them, I'm actually becoming more relaxed!

We might look to routines to make life 'safe', but we can't stress-proof our world. American journalist Scott Stossel appreciates this more than most. Stossel is a Harvard graduate, a celebrated author and a devoted dad. Yet fear rules his life. His phobias include: enclosed spaces, heights, fainting, being trapped far from home, germs, cheese, speaking in public, flying, vomiting and vomiting on airplanes. To overcome them, he's explored therapy, hypnosis, meditation, role-playing, eye-movement desensitization and reprocessing, self-help workbooks, massage therapy, acupuncture, yoga, Stoic philosophy, audiotapes and medication. So far, nothing has worked.[2]

Stossel has tried everything to make his world safe, yet he is still paralysed by anxiety. In contrast, the Bible speaks of Christians who faced unimaginable suffering yet were filled with peace. One of them was Paul. He writes, 'I have learned the secret of being content in any and every situation, whether well fed or hungry, whether living in plenty or in want' (Philippians 4:12). Reading this, we might assume that Paul had led a privileged life. But here's the reality:

> Five times I received from the Jews the forty lashes minus one. Three times I was beaten with rods, once I was pelted with stones, three times I was shipwrecked, I spent a night and a day in the open sea, I have been constantly on the move. I have been in danger from rivers, in danger from bandits, in danger from my fellow Jews, in danger from Gentiles; in danger in the city, in danger in the country, in danger at sea; and in danger from false believers. I have laboured and toiled and have often gone without sleep; I have known hunger and thirst and have often gone without food; I have been cold and naked. Besides

everything else, I face daily the pressure of my concern for all the churches.
(2 Corinthians 11:24–28)

Paul faces terrible trials, but he doesn't complain *or* boast in his own strength. Instead, he confesses that he came to the Corinthian church 'in weakness with great fear and trembling' (1 Corinthians 2:3). So what gives him such courage? He tells us in another letter: 'I can do all this through him who gives me strength' (Philippians 4:13).

In all of his suffering Paul relies on the power of Jesus. And in all our fear and weakness we can do the same. Instead of trying to make our world safe, we can trust in God to give us strength. And instead of retreating, we can step out in faith . . .

2. We risk in God's strength
Pastor and teacher John Piper says,

> On the far side of every risk – even if it results in death – the love of God triumphs. This is the faith that frees us to risk for the cause of God. It is not heroism, or lust for adventure, or courageous self-reliance, or efforts to earn God's favour. It is childlike faith in the triumph of God's love – that on the other side of all our risks, for the sake of righteousness, God will still be holding us. We will be eternally satisfied in Him. Nothing will have been wasted.[3]

Think of your favourite adventure film. What's the slogan? 'Explorer considers climbing a mountain, but opts instead for a nice cup of tea'? 'Young lawyer tackles corporate corruption, but can't be bothered with the paperwork'? I'm guessing not!

It's hard to reach out when we might be rejected. It's hard to try when we might not succeed. But God calls us to adventure, and some risks are worth taking. At the cross Jesus risked everything to save us, and he was killed. But through his death he redeemed the whole cosmos. Was it worth it? Yes! Godly risk is not about leaping into the unknown. It means entrusting ourselves to a God who holds us, no matter what.

When faced with a dilemma, I usually ask, 'What's the "safest" option?' or 'What feels most comfortable?' But there's a little verse in 1 Peter 3:6 that helps me to take a different approach: 'You are [Sarah's] daughters if you do what is right and do not give way to fear.'

These verses sound simple, but when we're torn between faith and fear, they cut straight to the core. Avoiding a difficult conversation? 'Don't be afraid and do what is right.' Scared to hand a relationship over to the Lord? 'Don't be afraid and do what is right.' Tempted to give in to an addiction? 'Don't be afraid and do what is right.' Instead of seeking comfort first, Peter teaches us to ask, 'What is right? Will this decision make me more like Jesus? Will it help or hinder others?' This is scary in the short term, but, ultimately, it's the path to peace and freedom. We might *feel* weak, but we can *trust* and then *act* on God's promises, instead of our feelings (Philippians 2:12–13). And as we do so, we will find that his word is stronger than our fears.

For those of us who naturally say 'no', Jesus calls us to risk. However, if we always say 'yes', then he teaches us something different: how to rest.

3. We rest in God's strength
Life can feel like an endless treadmill. But perhaps, like me, you're also scared of stepping off. When I stop, I think

about my feelings, my circumstances and my fears. I don't know how to manage them, so I stay busy instead. I tell myself, if I can just tick off my 'to-do' list, I'll have earned a sit-down. If I can just finish *this* task, I'll allow myself to rest. However, the lists never end. When one job is finished, another quickly takes its place.

Wouldn't it be wonderful to know that our work is done? Wouldn't it be wonderful finally to rest? This is what God offers his people. In fact, he insists on it! 'Remember the Sabbath day to keep it holy' (Exodus 20:8).

The world says, 'Work harder.' But God says, 'Rest.' And he leads by his example: 'By the seventh day God had finished the work he had been doing; so on the seventh day he rested from all his work' (Genesis 2:2).

This sounds good, but what does it look like in practice? An idyllic holiday away from the demands of life? A deep tissue massage or a good night's sleep? Not quite . . .

Think back to the Israelites, wandering in the desert. When they asked God for rest, he didn't reroute them to a spa retreat or parachute in some masseurs. He provided what they needed, but they stayed in the wilderness! That's because gospel rest is deeper than the absence of stress. Sometimes God answers our prayers by changing our circumstances; sometimes he answers them by helping us see old circumstances through new eyes.

We see this in the Corinthian church. Single people want to be married, married people want to be single, slaves want freedom, Jews want to become Gentiles and Gentiles want to become Jews (1 Corinthians 7). Everyone is discontented, but Paul offers some interesting advice: 'Be content and stay put,' he says (verses 17–20). If an opportunity for change comes up, you're free to take it (1 Corinthians 7:21, 28, 36), but in the meantime don't wish away your life!

We might feel 'useful' when we're busy, and 'useless' when we're still, but our identity is in Jesus, not in our diaries. Here's how 1 Corinthians 1:30 puts it: 'It is because of him that you are in Christ Jesus, who has become for us wisdom from God – that is, our righteousness, holiness and redemption.'

'Righteousness' is what tells God, the world and us that we are worthwhile. 'Holiness' is what makes us special and *different* from the world. 'Redemption' means 'freedom bought by a ransom payment'. These are amazing truths, but they cannot be earned. They are given to us already because we're in Christ.

Single or married, overworked or unemployed, joyful or despairing, in Christ, we are already worthwhile, already special and already free. So we can stop rushing around and we can trust in him to keep us safe.

Setting healthy boundaries

We can respond to anxiety by becoming walkovers (who say 'yes') or wall builders (who say 'no'). But as we walk in the light, we'll resist our fears.

If we're 'walkovers', then here are some reasons to say 'no' or 'not yet . . .':

1. If saying 'yes' reveals our desire to take the place of Jesus and 'rescue' others.
2. If saying 'yes' betrays a need to be needed.
3. If we think we're the only person who will do something 'right'.
4. If saying 'yes' takes away the opportunity for others to help.
5. If saying 'yes' creates an unhealthy dependence upon us (and not Jesus).

6. If saying 'yes' takes us away from greater needs
   (somewhere else).
7. If saying 'yes' keeps us from our real calling
   (and we're scared to step up).
8. If saying 'yes' keeps us from rest and stillness
   (and we're afraid to stop).
9. If 'yes' is a way of hiding behind tasks and keeping
   others at a distance.

If, however, we're natural wall builders, then here are some
reasons to say 'yes':

1. When 'no' is a way of avoiding relationship.
2. When 'no' is a cover for selfishness or fear.
3. When 'no' prevents us from serving God's people
   with our gifts.
4. When 'no' means that those weaker than us are
   asked to carry more.
5. When 'no' is our default answer, regardless of the
   question.
6. When there's no possibility of our 'no' ever
   becoming 'yes'.
7. When 'no' demonstrates unbelief in God's strength.
8. When 'no' is an excuse to avoid change.
9. When 'no' is a way of avoiding discomfort.

As Christians, our identity is rooted in Christ, not in what
we do – or avoid. This gives us the strength to go beyond
our instinctive 'yes' or 'no', and to ask deeper questions:
what does the Bible say on this issue? What opportunity
is being offered? Who (including me) will be blessed? As
we pray and seek God's wisdom, we're led by his love and
not by anxiety. This frees us to risk and to rest.

Thinking it through

Reread 1 Corinthians 1:30 and consider what it
means to be 'in Jesus'. How does this compare
to the slavery of 'keeping busy'?
If your response is always 'yes', then what lies behind
it? In what ways is God calling you to rest?
If your instinct is always 'no', then what are you
really trying to avoid? What risks are you avoiding
that need to be faced?
How can you move forwards? What needs to
change?

Handling panic attacks

When you start to panic, try not to fight it. Identify
the parts of your body that feel tense and then relax
them. Place the palm of your hand on your stomach
and breathe slowly and deeply (no more than twelve
breaths a minute). Breathe in for seven counts and out
for eleven. Repeat.

Stay in the situation and remind yourself that the
feelings will pass. Focus on what is going on around you
and keep going with what you were doing. When you
feel calmer, ask yourself these questions:

Is there any evidence that contradicts my panic?
What would I say to a friend who was thinking these
things?
What are the benefits and drawbacks of thinking in
this way?
How will I feel about this in six months' time?
Is there another way of looking at this situation?

When you feel anxious, write out a list of your concerns and pray through them, one by one. Cross out each item as you take it to God. Then tear up the piece of paper. Pick out some promises from Scripture that help to answer your fears. For example,

> The name of the LORD is a fortified tower;
>> the righteous run to it and are safe.
>
> (Proverbs 18:10)

Summary
We sometimes respond to anxiety by retreating or burning out. However, Jesus offers us a better way. In him we can risk and rest, knowing that we are already righteous, holy and redeemed.

A prayer for the anxious

Dear God,
I come before you at the start of this new day, feeling daunted and afraid. Thank you for listening. Thank you for promising to give me your peace.

Father, you tell us to bring our concerns to you. I list these before you now . . .

Please take these things upon your mighty shoulders. Forgive me for trying to carry them myself. Help me to trust them to you, and to rest in your strength.

Thank you that you are with me every moment of this day. Thank you for being my fortress, my anchor and my shield. Help me to go a step at a time, knowing that you are leading the way.
Amen.

We've brought our hunger and anxiety into the light. Next let's confront our need for control.

Gospel-shaped control

Here's a story about a little girl. It's her first day at nursery, and she's nervous and excited. She takes the teacher's hand and waves goodbye to her mum. They go to the playground. The girl walks past the swings to the sandpit. She stands at the edge, watching the other children as they throw sand, wrestle and squirm. Frowning, the little girl climbs in. Instead of playing, she makes her own space, smoothing the lines and warding off the messy kids. Why does she do this? Because she can't stop the mess elsewhere, but she can manage this one part. This bit is safe. This bit is *hers*.

The little girl becomes a teenager. She discovers other areas of life that she can't control. Her grandfather dies. Her family moves house. She is bullied at school.

She develops anorexia. Because she can't stop the mess elsewhere, but she can manage her body. This bit is *hers*.

She receives treatment. She eats more, but develops OCD. She scrubs her hands and she scrubs her room. Because she can't stop the mess elsewhere, but she can manage this one part. This bit is *hers*.

And as she grows, the pattern continues. It's less obvious, but the woman, Emma, still needs things to be done in a 'certain way'. Because she can't stop the mess elsewhere, but she can manage this one part. This bit is *hers*.

This is some of my story. But perhaps it's yours too? What's 'the mess' in your life? What are the things that you can't control? And what's the 'one part' you won't give up? The bit that's *yours?*

Like the girl in the sandpit, we invent rules to make life feel safe. But the more we try to keep them, the higher the standard becomes. Our rules rule us, until nothing but perfection is enough:

If I can't be the best, there's no point in trying.

I try to do everything absolutely perfectly so that no-one can be ashamed or shame me.

Perfectionism is sometimes seen as a positive character trait, but it's actually the very opposite of the gospel. Perfectionism tells me that if I do good things, I'll be accepted. The gospel says I'm accepted and *then* I do good.

Perfectionism doesn't allow for mistakes. But Christianity speaks of grace and the God of second, third and twenty-thousandth chances.

Perfectionism says we find freedom by taking control. But the gospel says that we find freedom by giving control to God.

Perfectionism says, 'Your best is never good enough.' The gospel says, 'Yes – and that's why Jesus died. Praise God!'

Perfectionism says, 'God can't be trusted.' The gospel says, 'No-one else can.'

Perfectionism says, 'If I'm not in charge, the world is in chaos.' The gospel says, 'God is in charge and he works all things for good' (Romans 8:28).

Perfectionism says, 'Try harder.' The gospel says, 'Rest.'

Perfectionism says, 'You can do it – and this is your hope.' The gospel says, 'You're helpless; but Jesus is your salvation.'

Christ in control

When I was threatened and afraid, anorexia seemed like a way of taking back control. However, it was 'self-control' that kept me enslaved!

> I'd tried to ring-fence my world with rules and rituals – systems to make life safe. But I'd never understood what it was to receive . . . in the past, I'd turned over a thousand new leaves. I'd made a hundred new beginnings, each doomed to failure. These resolutions were all about me – my rules, my strength, my gospel, my way. In the end, I lost all I tried to keep.[4]

Looking back, I can see that I've spent half of my life determined to take control and half of it determined to 'control' my control issues! Both are about fear (of being manipulated or abused) and pride (thinking that my way is best). But as I walk in the light, I have a new Lord, and his rule sets me free.

Worldly 'self-control' (like anorexia) is about bringing *my* desires under *my* will, through *my* strength. Gospel self-control is about bringing my desires under *Christ's* control, through *his* strength. With Christ's love, we're not bound by chains, but held close to his heart. Our battle is not to loosen those cords, but to recognize that they are 'cords of *love*' (Hosea 11:4).

Spirit-inspired control is not about 'taking ourselves in hand'. It's about handing our cares to a God who loves us more than we love ourselves. Nothing is outside *his* control (Hebrews 2:8), which means that he can be trusted to look after both the big things and the small. Every day we can bring these to him and trust him to be in charge.

Thinking it through

What areas do you 'need' to control?
Why is it hard to trust God with these things?
Are you in control of your life? Why/why not?
What does control promise to give you? What does
   it really deliver?
How is human self-control different from gospel
   self-control? (See Proverbs 25:28; 2 Timothy 1:7;
   1 Peter 4:7; 2 Peter 1:6.)
Psalm 91:1–2 says,

> Whoever dwells in the shelter of the Most High
>   will rest in the shadow of the Almighty.
> I will say of the LORD, 'He is my refuge and my fortress,
>   my God, in whom I trust.

How is the protection of the Lord described here?
   How has he demonstrated his ability to provide
   for you?

Challenging OCD

Dear Emma,
I read your blog post about having OCD. I check and count things, especially when I'm under pressure at work. I've prayed about it, but it's still hard, and I'm scared I'll forget to turn off the gas or make a terrible

---

mistake at work. It's also putting a strain on my marriage. What has helped you get better?
Craig

Dear Craig,
I'd love to say I'm completely 'better', but when I'm stressed, the old thoughts come creeping back. However, I'm learning not to act on them – which makes a big difference. Does anyone else know that you struggle with this? I would suggest going to see your GP, talking to a friend or leader at church and perhaps joining a support group for other sufferers (see e.g. http://www.ocduk.org/support-groups).

In terms of self-help, I try to remember that intrusive thoughts are just thoughts. God doesn't condemn me, and he's not surprised or shocked by them. Rather than trying to stop thinking them, I watch them, like they're on TV. I make a note of what they are, pass them to God and ask him to help me move on. This is difficult at first, but it gets easier with practice. In the short term it makes me more anxious, but it teaches me that I can feel uncomfortable or scared and not come to harm.

A friend who struggles with OCD gives this advice:

I came to see that 'spikes' (thoughts that come with fear, which said I had to do this or that, or own up to this or that, or prove this or that) did not have to be responded to. I would not be guilty if I ignored them. So I learned to let them come, let them hurt and let them pass, thereby learning that they were not really significant, but just 'thoughts'. Also it takes guts to stand up to the spikes – one commentator described it as getting into a swimming pool of ice cold water . . . [but] if you can hang on

> *in the pool for a minute or so, you realize you haven't died and*
> *that those thoughts were lies . . . This is how you learn that*
> *OCD can be broken, by experiencing the threat posed in your*
> *imagination/mind and deliberately standing against it.*
>
> Sin is bigger than us, and we can't choose to be perfect, no matter how hard we try. However, we don't need to get things 'right'. Jesus has kept the whole law perfectly, and we are in him. As we seek help and challenge our compulsions, he promises to help us and deliver us from our fears.
> Emma

Summary

When we try to take control, our rules become rulers and nothing is ever good enough. But Jesus is Lord, and his perfect love helps us to say 'no' to our compulsions and fears.

A prayer for the controller

Father,
Thank you that you rule the earth and nothing is out of
    your hands.
Thank you for your love and kindness. Thank you that
    I can give you all the concerns of this day, knowing
    that you will carry them.
I'm sorry for trying to run my life my own way. I'm sorry
    for trying to take your place and control my own
    world. I'm sorry that I don't trust you as I should.
    I'm sorry that I get caught up in rituals that only
    make me more stuck.

Please help me to live with fear and uncertainty.
Please help me to remember that the government
   is on your shoulders.
I give you my worries and receive your peace.
I give you my need to be perfect and receive your
   goodness.
I give you my rules and receive your grace.
I give you my busyness and receive your rest.
I give you my standards and receive your acceptance.
I give you my fears and receive your courage.
I give you my compulsions and receive your freedom.
Help me to step into this new day under your loving
   lordship and to trust my life to you.
In Jesus' name,
Amen.

Standing up to shame

Walking in the light means uncovering parts of our lives and history that we'd like to stay hidden. But we're not being exposed before critical eyes. In Jesus, we are righteous, holy and redeemed – set free from shame and from judgment. So let's consider how he redeems the past.

Most of us have scenarios in our history that we wish had never happened. Clocks we'd like to rewind, places we'd like to return to if only we could go over old ground and 'make it right'.

If you could turn back the clock, what would you change?

I would go back to age thirteen and stop myself from being sexually abused.

I would allow myself to mourn the death of my father and say that it is OK to grieve.

I would go back to age seventeen and tell myself that my mum did not mean to abandon me but that she was dealing with the death of her husband.

I would tell myself to stand up to the bullies, to stand up to my dad, and to tell myself that God loves me.

We can't reverse the past. So how can we work through our regrets? To answer, we'll need to sort through three powerful emotions: guilt, grief and shame. All three make us feel 'bad', but they come from different places, and each calls for a different response. We'll begin with guilt.

Grace for guilt

My eating disorder tore our family apart. Counsellors assured me that I was a good person in the grip of a sickness I couldn't control, but that wasn't the whole story. Once I'd reached my target weight, I went on hurting the people I loved, only in different ways. And I still do. Sometimes it's deliberate, and sometimes it's unintentional. Sometimes I feel guilty when I've done nothing wrong. At other times I can justify my behaviour, even though I've acted really badly. So how can I separate the truth from my feelings? By looking to God's Word for help.

The Bible talks about two kinds of guilt. First, there's godly sorrow that leads a person to repentance (2 Corinthians 7:10). This comes from the Holy Spirit, and it points us back to Jesus and the cross. Then there's another kind of guilt, which leads to condemnation and self-hatred. This comes from the devil, and it's utterly false.

False guilt is concerned not with failing God's standards, but failing my own. Maybe I want people to approve of me, but I have to make an unpopular decision. In my mind I'm convinced that the decision is right, but I feel 'guilty' that not everyone agrees. In all this I'm troubled by my feelings, not my conscience!

Real guilt is quite different. It comes from objective facts (e.g. God's Word) and points to concrete ways in which I've wronged God and others. With *true* guilt, I am driven *back* to the cross where only Jesus can pay for my sins. But then, in the assurance of forgiveness, the Spirit points me *forwards* to restoration. This is described in Joel 2:25, where God tells his people, 'I will make up to you for the years . . . eaten' (NASB). When we feel guilty, we want to make it up to God, but, amazingly, he promises to make it up to us!

We can't go back over our old mistakes and make them right, but Jesus already has. Through the cross he brings forgiveness for the past. And through the Spirit he redeems even our mistakes. We'll explore some of the ways he does this in the next chapter.

Thinking it through

What is the difference between true and false guilt? How does Jesus deal with both?
What are the regrets that you can't let go of?
How does the cross of Jesus offer you forgiveness for your mistakes?
How is the Spirit of Jesus reworking even your failures?

Grace for grief

It's easy to mix up guilt and grief. Both can paralyse us, lead to despair and make us feel that something is 'not right'. Sometimes what's not right is inside *us*. But sometimes what's 'not right' is out of our hands. In these situations we should feel 'sad' instead of 'bad'.

The Bible speaks about a good man called Job who loses all that he loves. Three of his 'friends' come to 'cheer him up', but then tell him he deserves his misfortune. No wonder they're called 'miserable comforters'. Yet, when faced with hardship, I sometimes talk to myself in the same way. 'Stupid me,' I say, 'I've brought this on myself.' But instead of feeling guilt, I should be feeling grief.

Grief is part of a broken world and we can't avoid it. Unfortunately, we often add to its weight. When we're grieving, we sometimes feel that we deserve to suffer or could have prevented it. When, for instance, someone takes their own life, loved ones often talk about feeling powerless, angry and *guilty*. 'I could have stopped it,' they say. 'I should have seen the signs.' This is false guilt and it makes our grief unbearable. It means that we spend our time and emotional energy feeling 'bad', when we need to feel 'sad' instead.

Managing grief

Common signs of grief include: numbness or disbelief, uncontrollable crying, feelings of guilt about surviving or not saying goodbye, trauma and emptiness. Allow yourself to feel these things, even at 'inappropriate' times, and ask for help. Keep going to church, meeting Christian friends, praying and reading your Bible.

It might feel difficult, but it's at times of loss that we need these things most.

Plan ahead for grief 'triggers' like anniversaries, holidays and milestones. If you're sharing a holiday or event with other relatives, talk to them about their expectations and agree on how you can best support one another.

Recognize that mourning is a process, and you can't speed it up. Consider different ways of remembering the person you lost, like making a scrapbook of memories, planting a tree, lighting a candle or praying with your minister.

In 1 Corinthians 15:26 death is described as our last enemy, so it's right that we should find it upsetting and unnatural. However, we don't mourn as those without hope. A time is coming when death will be crushed completely (1 Corinthians 15:25–26), and God promises to comfort us in our grief (Matthew 5:4). In time, he can even use our experiences to help others (2 Corinthians 1:3–4).

Thinking it through

When suffering, how are you tempted to blame yourself?

What grief are you carrying now? What false guilt are you struggling with alone? Ask Jesus to help you to share these and lay them before him.

In what ways have you known God's comfort? Thank him for his compassion and ask him to help you share it with others.

Grace for shame

Shame is often confused with guilt, but they are not the same thing. Guilt is about something we have *done* (our behaviour). Shame (a sense of painful exposure) is about who we *are*.

Shame can be a response to being hurt by others, for example through physical or sexual abuse. This means that we can feel shame when we have done absolutely nothing wrong.

In the next few pages we'll look at abuse and self-harm as sources of shame. We can only touch on this here, but you'll find more resources in the Appendix (pages 180–183), including an excellent series by Dan Allender called 'The Wounded Heart'.

Abuse

I was sexually abused, my father died when I was fifteen, and then my mother went to live with a new partner . . . I felt like I had been rejected, and this continued throughout my twenty-year (unhappy) marriage. I have therefore struggled with rejection issues and low self-esteem . . . I am trying to turn this around – I believe not in self-improvement, but in a God who can change me from the inside. It just seems to be a very slow journey!

I was attacked towards the beginning of the year. I was drinking myself into oblivion every night and self-harming terribly, trying to avoid the memories and flashbacks that I was getting, and all while trying to keep up with my teaching workload! There came a day when I was driving to school and something just snapped in me. I went into automatic mode, calmly drove myself to some shops, bought some rope and went

to a wood. I sat in the car for a very long time feeling the Lord's
eyes on me. Eventually I texted a friend and explained I needed
serious help. It was a big moment. I gave up trying to run my
life and keep up appearances. I gave in and admitted I was in
a bad way.

God hates abuse in all of its forms. He calls on his church
to protect and serve those in need (Isaiah 1:23; James
1:27), and condemns those who take advantage of the
'weak'. If abuse is part of your history, please know that
the Lord of heaven weeps with you. He has come to deal
with all kinds of darkness and he is gentle with those who
have been hurt.

If you have been abused, here are some truths to hold
on to:

God's love is not like the 'love' of your abuser.
    His love is safe and secure, and he promises that
    he will never harm us.
God will never take advantage of you or misuse his
    authority.
God is in control, not your emotions.
    As overwhelming as they seem, your feelings will
    not destroy you. God will help you to express them
    in safe places and with safe people.
God is just. He hates what has been done to you and
    he will punish those who have hurt you:

Therefore, this is what the LORD says:

    'See, I will defend your cause
        and avenge you.'
    (Jeremiah 51:36)

Whatever you have experienced,

You are not your past, nor what was done to you.
You were hurt, and *that* is wrong, not you.
Your abuse was not your fault.
You may feel shame, but it belongs to your abuser.
You and your body are precious and valuable.
You are not alone; other people can listen and help.

Abuse does not have to define you or your future. Please don't carry it alone:

Reach out – if you can speak to one or two people about your struggles, it helps. Be honest about how you are feeling and ask them to help you think about the way forward – how they might be able to support you, how your church might be able to support you, how your GP might be able to help. Hard and awkward and difficult as it is, things in the light are easier to bear than things in the dark.

(For more resources, see the Appendix, page 180.)

A prayer for the abused

Dear God,
Only you know how much I am hurting, and only you know what was done to me. I feel unclean, damaged and afraid. I feel like I'm lost in the dark.

Thank you that you understand. Thank you for washing away my shame. Thank you that you can heal what has been broken. Thank you that you give me courage to keep going. Thank you that you have good plans for me and my life. Help me to know these truths and to know your comfort. Help me to trust you to bring about justice. Help me to trust others again. Help me to hope. Bring me your wholeness and help me to know that the night is past.

In Jesus' name,

Amen.

Self-harm: a false covering for shame

Earlier in the book we thought about how Adam and Eve responded to shame. We saw that they lashed out and tried to cover themselves, and we've seen that we react in the same way. Self-harm can be one of the ways in which we try to cover our shame. It's a difficult pattern to break, but in the light of the gospel, we can find healthier ways to express how we feel.

In his book *Cutting* the counsellor Steven Levenkron encourages a self-harming patient (Simone) to speak her pain instead of writing it on her body. Here's part of their conversation:

'Maybe you need words instead of blades or knives.'

She looked confused, not understanding the comparison that I was making. 'How do words help the way you hurt?'

'Your words can build a bridge. Your bad feelings can travel over that bridge, away from you.'

'To what place?'

'To me.'

Simone was still puzzled. 'How can my bad feelings leave me and go to you? Then you will have bad feelings.'

'Your bad feelings don't have to hurt me. Maybe I will throw them away – something you can't do with them.'

'But I don't know you. How can this happen?'

'It can happen as you get to know me for a longer and longer time. Talking together will build the bridge.'[5]

This is not just a snapshot of a caring community. On a deeper level it's a picture of the cross. Jesus takes our shame and throws it away, for good (Romans 10:11). As he dies, our shame dies with him, and as he rises, he shares his glory with us.

When I was self-harming, I still remember the day when it occurred to me that the cross wasn't just something that was applicable to my life when I came to faith and I was then finished with it. I realized that the cross was how I kept going, how I was forgiven, what I lived in. It made a big difference to know that and to be able to fight with that truth in my mind.

As we bring our struggles into the light, we're able to challenge old beliefs and old patterns. We have a Saviour who covers our shame; which means that we can express our feelings in safe ways and with safe people.

Challenging self-harm

Dear Emma,
I want to stop cutting but I don't know how else to cope. I feel so ashamed of my scars, especially when it's hot outside and everyone else is in T-shirts. ☹
Jo

Dear Jo,
Thanks for writing. It's hard to make sense of our emotions, and cutting can seem like a release. But instead of trying to get rid of your feelings, what about looking at where they come from and what they are? This may sound scary, but your feelings can't hurt you.

They can be expressed in safe ways, without you harming yourself.

Here are some ideas:

Pray.

Write in a journal.

Listen to your favourite music and count the beats.

Colour in a colouring book.

Play your favourite instrument.

Tear up paper or pop some bubble wrap.

Use a red felt-tip pen to mark where you normally cut.

Tell one person how you feel.

Take a long hot bath and listen to your breathing.

Listen to music that expresses how you feel.

Rub ice across where you normally cut.

Rent your favourite film or read a book.

Go to a favourite 'safe' location (beach, park, woods, playground, etc.).

Put rubber bands on the places you cut, and 'ping' them instead.

Think of the advice you'd give someone else . . . and take it!

When you want to cut, pause, pray and then ask yourself these questions:

- Who can I call right now?
- How can I express my feelings in other ways: to God, friends or myself?
- Why do I feel I need to hurt myself? What has happened to make me feel like this?

- How will I feel when I am self-harming?
- How will I feel after hurting myself? How will I feel tomorrow morning?
- Can I get rid of the things I use to harm myself?
- Have I felt like this before? What helped me to deal with it? How did my feelings change?
- What has helped me in the past?

Self-harm can be a difficult pattern to break. But it is possible, especially with the right support. Have you told friends from church, your family or your GP? If not, I would really encourage you to do so, but there are also confidential helplines at websites, such as http://www.thesite.org.

You don't have to be ashamed of your scars, nor do you have to cover them. They're a reminder of hard times, but they're also proof that you're strong and have come through. If you don't want to discuss them, you don't have to! You can say nothing, or that they're from a while ago and you want to move on. There are also ways of making them less obvious, like over-the-counter creams, or 'camouflage' make-up (designed for this purpose). The charity Changing Faces provides information and runs clinics on skin camouflage (http://www.changingfaces.org.uk).

Blessings,

Emma

Summary

We've distinguished between guilt, grief and shame. Each causes us different kinds of pain, but Jesus brings healing for them all. For our guilt, he offers mercy and forgiveness.

For our grief, he brings comfort and hope. For our shame, he brings justice and healing.

A prayer for those who self-harm

Dear God,
I want to stop self-harming, but I don't know how. I feel
  trapped, but I want to be free. I'm ashamed, but I long
  to be loved.
Please help me.
Forgive me for treating my body harshly. Help me to see
  myself as you do and to take care of it.
When I'm frightened, hold me in your arms.
When I'm angry, grant me your peace.
When I want to harm myself, help me to stay safe.
Please help me to share my struggles with people who
  will help.
Help me to let go of my pain and to give it to you.
Help me to trust in your wounds and not in my own.
Cover my shame and lead me out of the dark.
In Jesus' name,
Amen.

We turn now to how the gospel speaks into our anger.

The antidote to anger

There are two ways that we naturally respond to anger: we express it or we suppress it.

When we express it, we say, 'I have the right to be angry. I'll pour it out and let it go – no matter whom it hurts.'

When we suppress it, we say, 'All anger is bad. So I'll pretend it's not there. I'll keep it hidden and I'll keep it in.'

Neither tactic helps.

Expressing our anger is like pouring petrol on a fire: it just stokes the flames. We're training ourselves to *feel* it, but not to deal with it.

Suppressing our anger is like seeing an engine light flashing on the dashboard but pretending it's not there. If we keep ignoring it, we'll eventually break down.

However, there's a third way to deal with our anger. The gospel says *confess* it. Take it to God and ask for his help. Find appropriate and safe ways to speak it out. Then resist it.

Confess it

Not all anger is obvious. But James tells us that it flows from deep wells:

> What causes fights and quarrels among you? Don't they come from your desires that battle within you? You desire but do not have, so you kill. You covet but you cannot get what you want, so you quarrel and fight. You do not have because you do not ask God.
> (James 4:1–2)

James starts by addressing 'quarrels' in church. Soon he is speaking about 'battles' and 'killing'. Why? Because, as Jesus says in Matthew 5:21–22, our anger is murderous. Or as we read in 1 John 3:15, 'Anyone who hates a brother or sister is a murderer, and you know that no murderer has eternal life residing in him.'

According to the Bible, we are angrier than we'd like to admit. Whether our anger explodes or implodes, it's like a grenade that's waiting to go off. So how can we dispose of it safely? By taking it to our Father in prayer. (See the prayer on page 136 for an example.) Only God can defuse our anger and bring us peace. He also teaches us to resist it.

Resist it

You might know the saying, 'Don't get mad, get even', but this is terrible advice. Getting even only makes us madder. The real antidote to anger is forgiveness. Jesus shows us the way in Matthew 5:39. He asks us to imagine that someone has struck us in the face. How might we respond? We could hide from our attacker (which allows them to bully us). Or we might punch back (which leads to more violence). In both instances anger takes the upper hand. To *resist* it, says Jesus, we must 'turn the other cheek' (Matthew 5:39).

Turning our cheek means answering anger with strength and with grace. It's about standing our ground, but offering our face and not our fist. Instead of sweeping sin under the carpet or running away, it means facing our hurts but refusing to pay them back.

This gracious response to those who hurt us is incredibly difficult. But the alternative is even worse. As American author Philip Yancey says,

> Not to forgive imprisons me in the past and locks out all potential for change. I thus yield control to another, my enemy, and doom myself to suffer the consequences of the wrong.[6]

However, let's be clear. Forgiveness is never about condoning wrongdoing or shutting our eyes to evil. By turning the other cheek, we never ignore evil or place ourselves or our loved ones in danger. If we're being abused, we stop the cycle of violence by withdrawing and calling on the appropriate authorities (e.g. church leaders and/or police). Shielded by our brothers and sisters, we face our attackers, as if to say, 'You wanted your anger to rule this situation. But grace will rule instead.'

There are times when we may need to seek legal protection. But for *all* wrongs we look forward to the perfect judgment of Christ. He sees and he will judge justly. This frees us to offer grace here and now (whatever society does with our abusers): 'Do not take revenge, my dear friends, but leave room for God's wrath, for it is written: "It is mine to avenge; I will repay," says the Lord' (Romans 12:19).

The greater debt

Walking in the light means walking free from anger, and we won't do this if we can't forgive. To help us, Jesus encourages us to put a figure on the debt we feel we are owed. In Matthew 18:21–35 he compares human bitterness to heaven's mercy, and tells a story like this:

Imagine that you've made some bad investments and owe £100 million. You've no hope of paying it back, but to your amazement the debt is wiped clean. You're celebrating when a friend approaches who owes *you* money (£3,000). How do you respond when that friend asks you for mercy? If you forget your own debt, you'll get angry. After all, £3,000 is quite a sum. However, if you compare it to what *you've* been pardoned, it is indeed a tiny amount.

When I'm wronged, I feel like I'm owed a million-pound debt. But Jesus helps me to have a sense of perspective. *My* sin against God is the real debt, not what's been done to me. So, before I cry out for 'justice', I need to ask God for forgiveness. Then, as *I* receive mercy from Jesus, I can start to pass it on.

Thinking it through

What makes you angry? Do you have the right to
   be angry?
Our anger can reveal a passion for *God's*
   righteousness, as well as our own. In what ways
   does your anger reveal a desire for justice? How can
   you pursue this through prayer and by working
   with others?
What sins do you need to ask forgiveness for (from
   God and from others)? Where do you need to offer
   forgiveness?
Using the Lord's Prayer as a model (Matthew 6:9–13),
   take these concerns to God. Focus on verse 12:
   'Forgive us our debts, as we also have forgiven our
   debtors.'

Challenging anger

Dear Emma,
I get so angry when I fail at a 'tiny task'. I simmer away
when I'm by myself, and then I hurt other people and
push them away. Have you any thoughts on how I can
calm down?
Fiona

Dear Fiona,
I'm afraid I can relate all too well to your 'simmering'. At
such times, we need to admit that we're angry and ask

---

for help. The first thing to do is to pray about it, and ask close friends for support. For example, 'I think I might struggle with anger – do you agree? How does it feel to be with me when I'm acting in this way? What can I do differently?'

Anger is a bit like a red light on the dashboard which points to deeper issues. We need to ask ourselves, what causes it? Does it mask other feelings, like embarrassment, insecurity, hurt, pride, shame or vulnerability? Take note of the times when anger has been an issue for you. Who have you been speaking to? What have you been reminded of? Where are your thoughts taking you?

On a practical level, be aware of your anger 'warning signs'. Monitor your anger and plot it on a scale from one to ten. Then, as the numbers rise, you can take action *before* you explode. Remove yourself from the situation if you can, and ask God to help you see events from a different perspective. These questions may help:

- How important is this in the grand scheme of things?
- Is it really worth getting angry about it?
- Is my response appropriate to the situation?
- Is there anything I can do about this situation?
- Picture your calmest friend. How would he or she respond?

It's important to admit our part in any arguments (Proverbs 28:13), but we should also be wise. Sometimes certain people are unsafe for us; we can forgive them, but we may have to set boundaries on our relationship.

Thank God for his grace in our simmering!

Emma

Summary

Anger is our natural response to exposure and hurt. But, by God's grace, we have choices about how to respond. Instead of expressing (boiling over) or suppressing our anger (quietly simmering), we can confess it. As we do so, we're reminded of God's justice and mercy. We receive his forgiveness and, through the Holy Spirit, we can begin to pass it on.

A prayer for the angry

Dear God,

I want to be calm, but I'm hurt and disappointed. I look around and I see injustice. Life seems so unfair!

Forgive me for taking matters into my own hands. Help me to trust in you to make things right.

I bring to you the people who have hurt me, and those whom I love. I bring to you the ways that I have hurt others. Please grant healing in these situations and help me to forgive.

When I'm angry, help me to look to you. Help me to step back and to calm down. Help me to know your mercy and your peace, and help me to show this to others.

In Jesus' name,

Amen

Let's bring the light of the new day to bear on our final struggle: despair.

Dealing with despair

When life is going well and we're settled and comfortable, it's easy to have hope. But when the light goes out or the brakes fail, when there's a stranger at the door or the phone rings in the middle of the night . . . that's when we ask big questions like these:

Is God big enough to handle floods or cancer?
How about divorce or bereavement?
Can he comfort those dealing with childlessness,
    suicide, grief and loneliness?
Can he take the weight of our despair?

To find answers, we can turn to a collection of 150 songs, right in the middle of the Bible. They're called 'Psalms', and here's a typical 'lyric':

I am overwhelmed with troubles
    and my life draws near to death.
(Psalm 88:3)

Our hymns are rarely so raw. Yet, in *God's* songbook, sorrow, anxiety and anger are common themes. Here even the heroes of faith can struggle with deep depression, and they are not condemned. In fact, they show us that despair can become worship when it is prayed.

Jesus demonstrates this on the night before he dies. Rather than denying his anguish, he prays it in the words of Psalm 88: 'My soul is overwhelmed with sorrow to the point of death' (Matthew 26:38). This is his act of worship, and it can be ours too. It's not about denying our pain, but looking to God in it and taking it to him. As we do so, we remember that he sees our pain and he has borne it.

Knowing Jesus, who has been through, and risen out of, the
darkness, gives me strength to carry on. I can't carry on in and

of myself, but he's promised to carry me through, and knowing that, I do.

Tempted to give up? Jesus cries, 'Why have you abandoned me?' Feeling bullied and persecuted? Jesus was hounded to the cross. Estranged from family and loved ones? Christ's own people rejected him. Desperate or over-whelmed? He asked, 'Is there any other way?' Jesus understands exactly what we're going through, *and* he shows us how to keep going. He teaches us how to speak out, and how to speak to, our despair.

Truth and tears

This is the subject of Tim Keller's eBook *The Grieving Sisters*[7] based on John 11. John tells us that Jesus' close friend Lazarus is dying – but Jesus doesn't go to him until it's too late. The dead man's sisters demand to know why he didn't arrive sooner. Jesus answers them, but he gives a very different response to each woman:

To Martha he says, 'I am the resurrection and the life. The one who believes in me will live, even though they die; and whoever lives by believing in me will never die. Do you believe this?' (John 11:25–26).

However, when Mary speaks, he simply weeps (verses 32–35).

One woman gets a Bible study; the other, raw emotion. Why? Keller explains that Jesus weeps for our suffering *and* he overcomes it. He answers grief with tears *and* with truth. Jesus shares our grief by weeping over death and confronting it as the enemy. But he also reminds us of the *truth*: that he has defeated death through his own death.

Right now Jesus is seated at the right hand of the Father, and one day soon he will return to this earth. He is our prize, and when he comes back, everything that is broken will be fixed (Revelation 21:5). Sorrow and mourning will disappear, and we will be filled with joy and gladness (Isaiah 51:11).

So then,

Praise be to the God and Father of our Lord Jesus Christ! In his great mercy he has given us new birth into a living hope through the resurrection of Jesus Christ from the dead, and into an inheritance that can never perish, spoil or fade. This inheritance is kept in heaven for you, who through faith are shielded by God's power until the coming of the salvation that is ready to be revealed in the last time. In all this you greatly rejoice, though now for a little while you may have had to suffer grief in all kinds of trials. These have come so that the proven genuineness of your faith – of greater worth than gold, which perishes even though refined by fire – may result in praise, glory and honour when Jesus Christ is revealed. Though you have not seen him, you love him; and even though you do not see him now, you believe in him and are filled with an inexpressible and glorious joy, for you are receiving the end result of your faith, the salvation of your souls.
(1 Peter 1:3–9)

How to keep going

Dear Emma,
Some days I don't want to get out of bed, and I can't see any hope for the future. I know that I have so much to

---

be grateful for, but I'm depressed and I can't see any way
out. At times I just want to give up.
James

Hi James,
Thank you for writing – that can't have been easy. You
don't mention if you have been clinically diagnosed with
depression, but if not, I would suggest visiting your
doctor, who will be able to rule out any underlying
physical causes and offer you a variety of options to help
you, including medication and different types of
therapy.

When I'm stuck and unable to see a way forward, my
friends tell me that *they* can. There's no shame in asking
for support – it's a vital step towards recovery –
especially because we can be so good at hiding our
problems from one another.

This doesn't mean sharing everything with everyone,
but being wise about which people we can trust. A friend
says this:

> Guard your heart and be discerning about who you share with –
> not everyone 'gets it', and when you're feeling rubbish, it's best
> not to have the people that don't get it doing you more damage.
> Gently mentioning the struggle, perhaps generically or
> abstractly, to see how someone responds can be helpful, or
> going to someone who you know has experience of struggling.

The Bible acknowledges the confusion and pain of life,
but it speaks into our sufferings with genuine hope. So
don't trust your feelings, and keep listening to God's
Word. The more we remind ourselves of the truth, the

more convinced we become of it – and even one simple verse can make a huge difference. This might mean inserting your name into Bible promises that speak about what you're facing ('To him who loves Emma and has freed her from her sins by his blood', Revelation 1:5), reading familiar passages in a different version of the Bible, or listening to favourite songs and hymns.

When we're depressed, it's easy to speak harshly to ourselves, but that only makes things worse. So be kind to yourself: by taking gentle exercise, eating regular balanced meals, getting to bed (and getting up!) at a reasonable time, or other activities that help you feel relaxed and cared for (like sitting in the sun).

You talk about giving up, but I'm not exactly sure what you mean. If you're feeling suicidal, then please do tell someone: a friend or loved one, your minister or a doctor. You can also call a helpline such as HopeLine UK (0800 068 4141). In Philippians 1:23–24 Paul says, 'I'm torn between two desires: I long to go and be with Christ, which would be far better for me. But for your sakes, it is better that I continue to live' (NLT). We might think it's better to be with Jesus, but it's important for our loved ones that we stay – and Jesus promises to help us. So please don't give up and don't battle alone.

There are mysteries around our suffering that we can't yet unpack. However, we don't have to figure them out or pray a certain amount for God to love us. Even when we let go of him, he has a firm hold of us. And he is at work, even when we don't feel it.

One of my favourite verses is from Hebrews 12:1: 'And let us run with perseverance the race marked out for us, fixing our eyes on Jesus, the pioneer and perfecter of faith.'

This verse compares the Christian life to running a race, and tells us to keep running, even when we're tired and losing heart. We do it by fixing our eyes on Jesus. He has marked out the race for us and he runs it perfectly. But he's more than just an example. The King James Bible describes Him as the 'author and finisher of our faith' (Hebrews 12:2) – in other words, he runs the race for us! This helps me to keep going, even when my strength runs out. And this is my prayer for you too. Emma

Thinking it through

How do the truths and tears of Jesus help you in your sadness?
Which people in your life can hope for you? What do they see that you're not seeing?
Read Psalm 43. This reminds us that even when we feel despairing, there is hope.

Summary

Even heroes of faith experience depression, but despair can become worship when it is 'prayed'. Weakness, then, is nothing to be ashamed of. In the midst of our needs we can look up to Jesus, look out to other believers and look forwards to the joy that is promised. This gives us an identity that goes far deeper than the labels we often assume. We are so much more than 'bulimic' or 'addicted' or 'depressed'. Before and beyond our struggles, we are 'in Christ'.

A prayer for the despairing

Dear God,
Thank you for being there for me, in good times and in bad.
I know that you love me, but right now I don't feel it. I feel
frightened and daunted by the day ahead.

When everything is dark, Lord, remind me of your
presence. When I'm numb and hurting, teach me to feel.
When I'm despairing, give me your hope. When I'm
exhausted, give me your strength.

Help me not to listen to lies. Forgive me for not trusting
you.

Thank you for protecting me and strengthening me. Lift
me from this depression and bring me close to you. Bring
others to help me and encourage me, and guard my heart
and my mind. Help me to do today in your strength.

In Jesus' name,
Amen.

We've revisited our old struggles in the light of the
morning. Now as we head towards the afternoon, we'll
explore what it means to keep walking 'in Christ'. One
word sums it up: 'Together!'

6 Afternoon
Sharing the light

When I was little and feeling frightened, I would hide in the bottom of the wardrobe. My mum would look for me and gently tap on the door. 'I'm fine in here,' I'd whisper. 'I like it in the dark.'

I didn't really like it. It was cold, and the dust made me sneeze.

She kept tapping, until eventually I opened the door. 'Come out,' she said, 'it's nice outside.'

I shook my head. 'It's much too bright. Why don't *you* come in here with *me*?'

'Because it's better out here. Your brother and sister are missing you. It's sunny and warm, and we want you with us.'

I wanted my mum to join me in the darkness, but she loved me by leading me out. We talked about the things I was scared of, and in the light my worries shrank. The monsters went back under the bed and the witches withdrew. Later, when my sister was frightened, I told her what Mum had told me. In this way, I shared the light with her too.

Jesus enters our darkness, but he doesn't leave us there, clutching a torch. He leads us into a family of light. Then he calls *us* to shine! He talks about this in Matthew chapter 5:

> You are the light of the world. A town built on a hill cannot be hidden. Neither do people light a lamp and put it under a bowl. Instead they put it on its stand, and it gives light to everyone in the house. In the same way, let your light shine before others, that they may see your good deeds and glorify your Father in heaven.
> (Matthew 5:14–16)

If we keep our faith to ourselves, it's like hiding our light under a bowl (or in a wardrobe!). Instead, we're saved to shine. Journalist Caitlin Moran talks about this in a moving letter to her daughter:

> Just resolve to shine, constantly and steadily, like a warm lamp in the corner, and people will want to move towards you in order to feel happy, and to read things more clearly. You will be bright and constant in a world of dark and flux, and this will save you the anxiety of other, ultimately less satisfying things like 'being cool', 'being more successful than everyone else' and 'being very thin'.[1]

As Moran says, our true calling is to 'shine, constantly and steadily . . . in a world of dark'. We do this, not by pretending to be *strong* or cool or clever or funny, but by being honest and real. Moran is not a Christian, but her words echo Matthew chapter 5. Jesus tells us we are a 'warm lamp in the corner'. He doesn't say, 'Burn brighter'; he simply tells us to clear away the obstructions and 'let it shine'. Shining is about sharing, not being 'cool, successful or thin'. It's about blessing one another.

So, as we come to the end of our day, we need to think about being a community of light. How do we share this light with the world? And how do we share it amongst ourselves?

We'll start by looking at the world beyond the church (its challenges and helps), and then we'll look at relationships within the church.

The world

As churches, we may feel equipped to handle 'spiritual' stuff (like Bible studies), but what about mental illness?

How do we help those amongst us who are alcoholic, self-harming, suicidal, phobic, traumatized or chronically ill? Can we deal with these issues in-house? Or should we call in the experts?

Both.

We know by now that Jesus is Lord over body, mind and soul. But while *Jesus* has these things covered, we Christians may not. The average church leader will not be equipped to deal with a psychotic episode, and they can't prescribe or manage medication. At points like these we need professional help.

So how do we integrate professionals within the life of the church? Here's an illustration.

Shepherds and vets

In the Bible church leaders are described as shepherds over their flock (e.g. 1 Peter 5:2). They're in charge, but when their sheep become sick, they seek specific expertise. They take them to the vet.

Are the shepherds and the vets in opposition? Absolutely not! They're partners, and neither feels threatened by the other. The shepherd is grateful for the vet's knowledge and follows his advice. Yet, while the vet often helps for a limited period, the shepherd remains. He cares for his sheep in sickness *and* in health.

There are situations where, as churches, we need specialist support (e.g. when dealing with psychosis or schizophrenia). In these instances sufferers may be under the care of 'vets' for their whole lives. But even here the church continues to shepherd its flock. We support each other *through* treatment – as we care for anyone who's sick. This includes visiting one another in hospital, praying, talking through treatment options and providing practical or financial assistance. Alongside medical care, we continue to provide soul care.

In a moment we'll see how churches can help their sick 'sheep'. But before we do, let's consider the 'vets'. How should we assess the 'professional' care on offer? After all, we don't defer to everyone in a white coat. We spend time researching them, and we look for qualifications and recommendations. And as we do, here are some issues that may be worth thinking through.

Getting a diagnosis

Dear Emma,

For a while now I've been feeling very low and worrying about even the tiniest things. I don't want to talk to my friends, as they won't understand. Do you think I should go to the doctor? I'm scared he'll tell me I've got something bad, or that my boss will find out. And I don't want to be labelled.

Jess

Dear Jess,

Thanks for writing. I don't think I've got 'the answer' for you, but here are some thoughts.

Sometimes having the courage to speak out can help us feel more accepted by others. I know it's scary, but I really think that telling one or two others will make a difference. Even if you get a negative reaction, you don't have to keep things hidden any more. And your honesty might help others to share their own experiences. I found it useful to talk about my depression, as friends could see it more clearly than me, and they were able to give me practical and emotional support. But it's up to you. What I would say is, if you don't talk to a friend, you should speak to a professional so you're not on your own.

When we're struggling, our GP (General Practitioner) can be a great source of support. GPs work in partnership with other medical professionals and will refer us if they can't treat our problem themselves. It's worth asking if any doctors at your practice specialize in mental health. Remember that they should be professional and supportive: if they're not, then ask to see someone else or change practice.

In terms of getting a diagnosis, there are pros and cons. If we're diagnosed with something concrete, it can help us (and others) to understand why we find certain things difficult or behave the way we do. Once something has a name, we can find out more about it and maybe treat it. (There are also illnesses like certain kinds of bipolar disorder that need medication.)

Remember that when you speak to your GP or medical professional, it's in confidence, so they won't share what you tell them with your boss or others. They may suggest lifestyle changes or offer you medication, counselling or cognitive behavioural therapy (CBT). This looks at why we think and act the way we do, so that we can identify problem areas and challenge unhelpful beliefs and behaviours.

Another plus is that having a label can remind us not to rely on our feelings (especially when they tell us lies like 'I'm not sick' or 'I don't deserve help'). Naming our struggles can help us rely more on God and his people, and once they're identified, we may feel less ashamed of them. Having a diagnosis can also be a way of meeting others in similar situations (e.g. at support groups).

This said, there are negatives too. Sometimes having a label can squash my hopes for recovery, or just the opposite: it can raise my hopes for an easy solution that might not be there. It can become my identity or an excuse for things that aren't affected by it. For example, I may become over-dependent on other people when

I'm capable of doing some things myself. It might
also change how they see me or how I see them. They
might think of me as uniquely 'broken', and I might be
tempted to see them as 'fixers'!

It's always tempting to look for a programme for
rescue, instead of Jesus, and this can also apply to
medication. While some medications are essential,
others can become 'the whole answer', instead of a way
of tackling underlying issues.

These are some of my thoughts. If you can, talk to
your church leaders or friends: God gives us others so
that we don't suffer alone.

In Jesus,

Emma

Medication

Mental illness is a broad term for a variety of disorders
in different categories. Some, like schizophrenia, have
such a strong biological component that medications are
essential. (Over 70% of people with psychosis or schizophrenia will benefit significantly from antipsychotic
medication. The remaining 30% will benefit in part, and
would be extremely unwell with no medication.[2])

There are four main types of psychiatric medications
listed in the British National Formulary: antipsychotics
(for psychotic illnesses like schizophrenia), antidepressants, mood stabilizers (for bipolar affective disorder)
and hypnotics and anxiolytics (which don't treat active
illness but can help with symptoms, usually in the short
term).

We can't cover them all, but let's consider one of the
most common types: anti-depressants.

Antidepressants

Dear Emma,
Should I go on antidepressants? Will they alter my
personality? Have you ever tried them, and did they
help?
Ian

Hi Ian,
Antidepressants work by balancing chemicals in the
brain (neurotransmitters), which affect mood and
emotions. They don't make you 'happy', but they're not
meant to do so. When they work, they help to bring
you closer to your normal self. This might be someone
bursting with life and positivity. But it's equally likely
to be a very human mixture of sadness, hope, despair,
longing, confusion and all kinds of other emotions that
'happy' doesn't describe.

There are different kinds of antidepressants, and they
will suit different people with different needs. Doctors
usually start patients off on a fairly low dose, which may
need to be adjusted before you see any effects. Give them
time. Some medications start by working gradually, and
your loved ones may spot the signs of improvement long
before you do.

Research suggests that after three months of
treatment, around 50–65% of people with moderately
severe depression will be much improved. However, it
can take a while to get the right dosage for you. For this
reason it's recommended that you keep taking
prescribed medication for at least six months after you
start to feel better.

The first antidepressants I tried made me feel sick and permanently groggy. However, when I changed medication, I noticed a big improvement. So if you're having problems, or the tablets aren't helping, go back to your GP.

Here are some questions you could ask:

What type of depression/sickness do I have and how serious is it?

What treatment options are available?

What should I do if I'm in a crisis, feel suicidal or need emergency help?

What type of drug are you prescribing, and how does it work?

Are these drugs addictive, and if so, are there alternatives?

Could they interfere with any of my other medications?

What are the associated side effects?

When will they take effect and how will I know?

How long will I need to take them for?

I'm thankful for the ways in which professionals and prescribed medication have helped me. But in my experience, they're just part of the solution. Mental illness can point to other areas of our lives that need to be reassessed, such as lifestyle choices, ingrained patterns of thinking and acting, ways of handling emotions, or unresolved tensions in relationships or work. This is where counselling can be a help.

Emma

Counselling

Counselling is a talking therapy where people can share their struggles in a confidential environment. This may happen face to face, individually or in a group, over the phone, or by email or Skype. It can last for a single session or continue over many years, although it's normally time-limited. During this period all sorts of issues may be covered, from early childhood to future fears. Many of these are painful, but the goal is for those unpleasant feelings to be processed and understood so that they stop interfering with daily life.

Provided that we do our research, counselling can be an important source of support. The ideal scenario is to work with Christians who have professional training. This, however, is not always an option, and even where it is, we need to be cautious. It makes sense to use counsellors from an accredited register, for example the Association of Christian Counsellors (http://www.acc-uk.org). However, be aware that their approaches may differ, and it might take a while to find someone who fits your needs.

Speaking personally

When I was treated for anorexia, Glen and I searched on both sides of the Atlantic for support. Some counsellors refused to talk about God at all, and others suggested I might be demon possessed. When we finally found a qualified pastor with thirty years of experience, he said that my problems were too big. I left his office in despair, thinking, 'The NHS can handle me, but God thinks I'm too much!'

On the other hand, I've had a couple of Christian counsellors who have helped me enormously. They've showed me God's love in a very concrete sense and corrected areas where I had a wrong view of God and of myself. Together, we acknowledged that Jesus was with us and, as we parted, we acknowledged that he went with us too. They helped me love Jesus more – and this equipped me for every challenge, not just the ones we discussed. Most importantly, I learned to rely upon God, instead of upon them or myself.

If you're referred through the NHS, then Christian counselling may not be an option. But secular counselling can be helpful too, as long as we think it through. In the same way that we would weigh the advice of a good non-Christian friend, so we'll want to process our counsellor's words according to our gospel beliefs. Much of what is said will be very helpful, but some may need to be questioned or reframed with reference to biblical teaching (see the letter to Lizzie below).

Dear Emma,
My GP has referred me for counselling. I can't afford to go privately, and I really need some help. But I talked to a friend and he said it wouldn't be right to see a non-Christian. What do you think?
Lizzie

Hi Lizzie,
In my view, there's no 'one-size-fits-all' answer, I don't think. Secular counselling *can* be useful, but we need to approach it thoughtfully and prayerfully. My feeling is that 'it's good to talk', but at the same time, it's essential to be discerning in how we *listen*. Here are some questions you might want to ask:

---

1. What approach do you take to counselling? What training do you have?
2. What experience do you have of helping people like me?
3. I'm a Christian. How will you work with my faith?
4. What would a typical counselling session involve, and how much will it cost?
5. How many sessions do you usually recommend?

If you decide to pursue secular counselling, don't leave your faith at the door. Be frank about your beliefs, filter what you hear through the Bible's teaching and, outside the sessions, talk things through with a mature believer.

Do ask your therapist to work with your beliefs. Practitioners may not share them, but they are meant to work *with*, rather than against, your faith. When I was up front with a non-Christian counsellor, it was a big help. In one session, for example, we were looking at building self-esteem. My counsellor said that I was a good person and should love myself more. I explained that the Bible teaches that we're not naturally good, but that Jesus forgives our sin and welcomes us anyway. So, instead of giving me affirmations like 'I'm a nice person; I deserve to be happy', we picked out Bible verses that talked about forgiveness and our value in Jesus. We achieved her aim – to stop me from condemning myself – but we based it in Bible truths, not just positive thinking.

Counselling *can* be used by God, but remember, he transforms us through his Word and through his people. Whatever you decide, make sure that these foundations are firmly in place.

Yours,

Emma

Carrying one another

If you're struggling with mental illness and you go to your GP, you're being enormously brave. You're making yourself vulnerable. You're saying no to a host of voices that tell you, 'You're not sick enough; you don't deserve any help.'

The last thing you want to hear from your GP are those very words: 'I'm sorry, but you're not ill enough to qualify for treatment.' Yet for one in eight children with a 'life-threatening condition' (like severe anorexia), this is actually what happens. Our health care system is overburdened, and even for the 'lucky' ones (who qualify for treatment), there's an average waiting time of 110 days.[3]

110 days to lose more weight.
110 days of fighting and pleading and weeping and
    despairing.
110 days to move from 'life-threatening' to 'life-
    ending'.
110 days to move from wanting help to no longer
    caring.

I know this, because it's happened to me – twice.

The first time I was thirteen. My mum noticed that I was losing weight and dragged me to the doctor. There was a long queue in the surgery, and the doctor seemed distracted. He rolled up my sleeve: 'Not much of you, is there? I take it you're eating enough?'

I mumbled that it was hard, but he nodded before I'd finished and turned to my mum: 'Look, she's a teenager. Her body's changing, and it's not unusual to have irregular periods. It's nothing that a good night's sleep and some exercise won't sort out.' And that was that.

Four months later I could barely speak, let alone run. My cheeks were sunken, and I was permanently cold. People were noticing that something was wrong. But I no longer cared. We made an emergency appointment with a different doctor. This one said, 'You need treatment now. In another week it'll be too late.'

That was the first time. The second time I was in my twenties, and I made an appointment for myself. Burning with shame, I tried to explain. 'I've got a history of anorexia.' I cleared my throat. 'And I think – I think, it's starting up again.'

The doctor examined me. 'You can't afford to lose more weight,' she said. 'I'll refer you to a specialist treatment centre – but I must warn you, the waiting lists are con-siderable. I don't think you're thin enough to qualify.'

A few months later I received an appointment for the eating disorders wing of a local hospital. By that stage my weight had plummeted further. They said I still wasn't sick enough for in-patient care. 'Come back in a month's time,' they said, 'and we'll monitor your progress.' (Subtext: 'We'll help you if you lose more weight.')

Four weeks later I finally qualified for care. But I no longer wanted to be helped.

None of this is about pointing the finger or apportioning blame. The system is overstretched and under-resourced. Doctors can refer you, but they can't make beds where none is available. And treatment centres have to take the most critically ill patients (unless you can afford to pay for yourself). Nonetheless, the earlier patients receive treatment, the higher their likelihood is of recovery.

Although we might value the professionals highly, they cannot provide all the care that we need. And it's not just children with eating disorders who need help. In the NHS more than one in ten patients waits over a year just to be offered an assessment for their mental health problem, and one in six has attempted suicide while waiting.[4]

As a church, we can't force an anorexic to eat, stop a self-harmer from cutting, or lift a life-threatening depression. But working in partnership with mental health services, we can minister to those who suffer. We can support patients/carers and provide practical and emotional support. We can step forward where the system struggles.

Perhaps you're a Christian seeking medical or psychological help, for yourself or for others. You may feel like you have nothing to offer in comparison with 'the professionals'. But consider this:

110 days of prayer, compared with 110 days of
  waiting.
110 days of support, compared with 110 days of
  feeling alone.
110 days of Christlike love, compared with 110 days
  of growing despair.

I remember a friend, when I first told him my story, just holding me and crying with me, and I'll never forget that. He was willing to hold some of my pain as my brother, and that gave me courage to stand.

As churches, we work with professionals and are grateful for their expertise. But our hope runs deeper than treatment plans and medication, and our concern extends to heart and soul as well as body and mind.

We are there before the emergency services step in, and we continue to care after they've gone. We do this by praying, loving and pointing one another to Christ. In his strength we hold each other's pain, and we give one another courage to stand. This is how we live as a community of light.

Relationships within the church

Sharing the light

We've seen that there's a place for doctors, therapists and medication, but we've also seen the limitations of such help. Now, as we think of our relationships in the church, we enter the heart of soul care. This is summarized by Paul in his letter to the Galatians: 'Carry each other's burdens, and in this way you will fulfil the law of Christ' (Galatians 6:2).

Paul doesn't say, 'Carry some people's burdens' or 'Carry the burdens of the especially weak.' He says, 'Carry each other's burdens.' God has designed us to depend on each other – and no-one is exempt. Here are some words from Bible teacher John Stott:

> God's design for our life is that we should become dependent on him and on one another . . . we are all designed to be a burden to others. You are designed to be a burden to me and I am designed to be a burden to you. And the life of the family, including the life of the local church family, should be one of 'mutual burdensomeness'.[5]

How do you feel about being called 'a burden'? Frankly, I hate it. I don't want to be a bother and feel bad when others have to step in. To meet the deadline for this book, I've had to ask for help with babysitting, and I found that a challenge. But if I think like this, I lose sight of something very important: my salvation! The profoundest fact about me is that I *am* a burden. Jesus has to rescue me, and he's glad to do it. If I can't let others carry me, I'm forgetting who I am. I'm called to be carried – and I'm called to carry others too.

How do you feel about *carrying* other people's burdens? Perhaps you've fought for your own independence and expect others to do the same. Again, if we think like this, we forget who we are. Church is not a club for individual Christians, but a body of interdependent parts. We need one another! This week my friends have lifted me, but later I hope I can do the same for them. And as we serve one another, each of us is blessed.

In a letter to her church one woman explains what it means for her to be 'carried':

I have a confession to make. I have been diagnosed with a mental health illness. The question is, will you now walk on the other side of the road?

It is not easy for me to admit I have a problem, namely because of the stigma, and because society is less accepting of a mental illness than of a physical illness. Secondly, I am a Christian and I feel that somehow Christians should be immune from mental health issues. I'm not sure if this is a view shared by others.

In March I was diagnosed with atypical anorexia nervosa . . . I was under severe pressure at work and at home, and I felt that life was getting out of control. Unfortunately, instead of asking for God's help, I found something I could control – my diet. I refused to listen to family and friends until I realized that I was in danger of starving myself to death. At that point I was admitted to the Priory, where the long road to recovery began. It was at that point that I allowed God to take control of my past, present and future.

I stayed in hospital for two months, and with God's help and the support of friends and family, I am on the road to recovery. Yes, I am still mentally fragile, and yes, I am struggling still. I am indebted to those people who have supported me and not judged me harshly.

I was really helped by 1 Peter 5.10: 'He will restore, support, and strengthen you' (NLT).

One day I will be strong again, but until then, please don't walk on the other side of the road.

Everyone who suffers from a mental illness needs your love and support. There but for the grace of God go I.

The phrase, 'walking on the other side of the road', comes from the story of the Good Samaritan (Luke 10:25–37). A traveller is beaten, stripped of his clothing and robbed. First a priest and then a Levite pass him by. Finally, a Samaritan shows up. Jews and Samaritans were enemies, but the Good Samaritan 'came where the man was, and when he saw him, he took pity on him' (Luke 10:33). The Samaritan shows us what it is to love one another – by drawing near (not walking by), seeing pain (not closing our eyes to it), and showing compassion (not shutting off). We might feel underequipped and we might not know exactly what to do or say. But by refusing to 'walk on the other side of the road', we can be a community of burden bearers – stumbling, but lifting one another to the light.

After Jesus describes the Good Samaritan, he says to his listeners, 'Go and do likewise' (Luke 10:37). Every one of us is asked to draw near, to see and to show compassion. What's your response to this call? Maybe you're enthusiastic in theory, but would like a bit more guidance.

Or perhaps you've tried to be a Good Samaritan, and it hasn't seemed to work. To finish this section, I've included two letters. In the first I give practical advice for those who want to help, and in the second I talk about our limits as helpers and the need to balance realism and hope. At different points we will need to hear both messages.

Caring for your flock

Dear Emma,
I'm on the leadership team of a church in the city.
We want to be a place where everyone feels welcome,
especially those who are going through hard times.
Have you any advice on how to do this?
Graeme

Dear Graeme,
It's great that you're thinking in these terms. In my
view, leaders need to be talking about mental health,
both informally and from the pulpit. Instead of just
telling people to 'trust God', show your congregation
how to develop practices that will help them to grow
in their faith. This means modelling weakness, and
challenging the belief that Christian leaders must be
strong, extroverted and 'together'. It's also vital to train
and equip the church family on mental and emotional
health – for example the value of rest, the dangers of
perfectionism, the importance of vulnerability and the
value of community.

We should expect mental health struggles (both in
our congregations *and* in our teams). And, as churches,
we mustn't assume that mental illness is simply caused

---

by sin (though sins will play a part). What I mean is this: we live in a fallen world. Much of our suffering – including mental ill health – has come about through no fault of our own. At the same time, since the fall sin permeates everything – from raising children, to serving in church, from our bodies to our minds (including mental health). This means that there is sin involved in how we respond to mental illness, just as there is in how we handle physical illness. For example, if I break my leg, this is not 'sin'. But there *can* be sin in the ways in which I respond to my pain. In the same way, anxiety, for example, is not sin – but I can sin in the ways that I respond to it.

Whatever we face, we're all sinners and we're all trying to become more like Jesus. It's worth explaining this as part of a church statement of belief. Reinforce the fact that mental illness does not mean we are uniquely sinful or lacking in faith! Back it up with a clear and consistent pastoral support strategy, and ensure that people know whom to approach for help within the church and beyond (e.g. by providing links to helpful organizations).

With sufferers, I think the main thing is to keep praying and to be there for them long term. Don't be frightened of mental illness, but do take time to find out more about it, ask how it feels and if/how you can help. Allow God to work in ways other than sudden, instantaneous recovery, and invite testimonies from those who aren't necessarily free from struggles, but are working them through. Reincorporate sufferers into community, for example by building confidence and helping them to use their gifts (especially in small and

pressure-free environments). Provide space for
different needs, and think of offering community
beyond Sundays. This might mean providing room for
people to pray and sit in silence, having someone on a
help desk who is trained to listen, and offering different
kinds of worship, opportunities to talk in private after
services and visits for those who can't get to church.

Above all else, remind your people that they are
valued and valuable, and keep pointing them back to
Jesus and his grace. It sounds like you are doing this
already; which is wonderful to hear.
Emma

Dear Emma,
My best friend is struggling with an eating disorder.
I've given her Bible verses about honouring her body,
but she's getting worse. I feel like what I say makes no
difference. How can I get her to start eating?
Judy

Dear Judy,
Every fibre of me wants to say, 'Here's the answer.' But
I can't, because there is no fix, at least, not in human
terms. Practical advice and shared experiences are
helpful, but in themselves they're not enough. Not
enough to change the heart of whoever is struggling,
and therefore, not enough to change their struggle.

I'm not enough – and neither are you. We can't climb
inside another person's head and heart, and we can't
change our own. You can encourage your friend and pray
for her, and that's huge – but you can't make her eat. So

please, don't give up on being her friend, but do give up on being her saviour.

None of us can save another person, which is why we need Jesus. He is the heart of our faith, and only he can change your friend's heart. This is her hope, and it's our hope too. I've sent you some links and practical advice (see the Appendix), which may help. However, your greatest need (and your friend's) is to stay close to him. How is your own walk with Jesus going? Are there others in your life encouraging you? It's hard to love someone who's in pain, and it's important that you're being spiritually fed yourself.

I heard a minister describe the work of encouragement as acting like a sheepdog. Jesus is the real Good Shepherd, and we just nudge other lost sheep closer to him. I hope you don't mind me saying this, but it sounds to me like you're being a faithful sheepdog. You're doing what you can, and Jesus sees this. But there are limits to how much you can help – you are not the Good Shepherd – only Jesus is.

I understand that you feel powerless, and you're searching for answers. But keep looking to Jesus and don't despair. God's power is made perfect in our weakness. He hears you, he loves you, he loves your friend and, in the end, he will work all things for good. With love,
Emma

Judy's experience of powerlessness is so familiar in pastoral care. At times we all feel helpless in the face of problems that simply won't shift. We are desperate to help, and yet incapable of making things better. This is frustrating, to say the least. Ironically, though, it's in our experiences of brokenness that God shows up in the most powerful ways. In fact, it's precisely as we feel our weakness that God works in strength.

A community of wounded healers: scar stories

When I look across the pews on a Sunday morning, other people seem happy, balanced and together. However, from the outside, perhaps I seem healthy too. *I* know I'm not, and I've got the scars to prove it. But I try to keep them hidden. They're ugly and shameful. I don't want them to be seen!

But what if it wasn't just me? In fact, what if I discovered that *everyone* was scarred? How would this change the way that I relate to others? Would I still feel frightened and ashamed? Or would I start to open up? Theologian Henri Nouwen says,

> We all are wounded people. The main question is not, 'How can we hide our wounds?' so we don't have to be embarrassed, but, 'How can we put our woundedness in the service of others?' When our wounds cease to be a source of shame, and become a source of healing, we have become wounded healers.[6]

Nouwen tells us that everyone has scar stories. Often we're embarrassed by them and try to hide. However, when we share them instead of covering them up, something remarkable occurs. Our scar stories can become a source of healing instead of a source of shame.

It sounds amazing, doesn't it? But how is this possible? How do we move from hating our struggles, to owning them and using them to bless others?

The Bible says that it happens when we meet the Healer who touches us with his own pierced hands. Jesus shows us his wounds and is not ashamed. He speaks to us softly and says, 'Let me tell you the ultimate scar story: mine.'

Surely he took up our pain
   and bore our suffering,
yet we considered him punished by God,
   stricken by him, and afflicted.
But he was pierced for our transgressions,
   he was crushed for our iniquities;
the punishment that brought us peace was on him,
   and by his wounds we are healed.
(Isaiah 53:4–5)

This is my testimony. I came to Jesus with my scars and my shame. He took them and gave me a new story, one that needed to be told. I was scared to share it, but as I did, something amazing happened. People answered.

'You're not alone,' they said. 'Keep talking.'

Since then I haven't stopped. God is using my scars – and he will use yours too.

It started with an invitation to speak at a training day for youth leaders. The topic was 'Eating Disorders from a Sufferer's Perspective', and I was asked if I could help. I wanted to hide, but I felt that God was asking me to speak from the heart. So I got up and told my story.

'Hello. My name's Emma, and twice in my life I've suffered with life-threatening anorexia.'

With my head bowed, I spoke before an audience of strangers. I expected disapproval and disgust, but they held my words like they were precious jewels. Some nodded, and others had to translate my struggles into their own – but no-one scoffed. They spoke of their own grief and even wept for mine. And as we talked about God's kindness, there was beauty, even in our mess.

Moved by this experience, I decided to start a blog. At first I wrote for those with anorexia, but I was startled by the response. Many who replied had never had eating disorders, but could identify with my experience. I heard from men and women, young and old, married and single, gay and straight, those who led churches and those who were frightened to enter them.

'Keep talking,' they said. So I did.

I wrote a book called *A New Name*. On the cover was a picture of my face, with the word 'anorexia' inscribed underneath. Inside I penned a picture of my heart, in all its ugliness and mess. I was stunned when others said, 'Me too'.

More speaking invitations followed. These ranged from breakfasts in church halls, to addresses on floodlit stages. I didn't offer solutions or brilliant advice; I simply went first and shared my scars. Often the real work happened at the end of the event. One by one, people would come forward and tell their own scar stories . . .

An ex-drug addict who'd just got out of prison.
A man of my father's age, with tears streaming down his face.
A single mum.
A church leader struggling with depression.
A boy who was being bullied at school.

As I spoke of Christ's beauty and my mess, they said, 'I've never had an eating disorder. But your story is my story too.'

It's hard to open up and show our scars. However, when we do so, we start a conversation. We say to one another, 'I understand, because I'm like you.' It's not because I have an eating disorder or struggles with my mental health. It's because I'm human. I'm hungry and anxious and controlling and ashamed and angry and sad. I'm sinful. And the cry of my heart is to know that you are too.

German pastor and theologian, Dietrich Bonhoeffer, puts this beautifully:

> Anybody who has once been horrified by the dreadfulness of his own sin that nailed Jesus to the Cross will no longer be horrified by even the rankest sins of a brother . . . Worldly wisdom knows what distress and weakness and failure are, but it does not know the godlessness of man. And so it also does not know that man is destroyed only by his sin and can be healed only by forgiveness. Only the Christian knows this. *In the presence of a psychiatrist I can only be a sick man; in the presence of a Christian brother I can dare to be a sinner.*[7]

Nothing is more powerful than seeing myself in the face of another. Nothing is more powerful than hearing the words: 'Me too'. But as we share our scars, we point to the light outside of us. We say to one another, 'Don't be ashamed. I'm also a sinner. But look, isn't *he* beautiful? He will heal us. He will take away our sin.'

I spoke about this recently, and afterwards a woman approached me. For the first twenty minutes she said nothing, because she was bent double weeping. Finally, she spoke. She said, 'The darkness in you is also in me. But it's the first time I've heard someone speak of it. I go to church, and everyone seems happy. I pretend I'm happy too. But I'm not. I'm sad and ashamed. Today I heard you and I thought, if she can say it, I can say it too. I want to know about this Jesus. I want to stop being ashamed.'

When we dare to be sinners in front of one another, something wonderful happens. We come together, not as the healthy versus the sick, but as needy sinners who are united by God's grace. This means that when you ask me how I'm doing, I can afford to be honest. When I'm slipping into darkness, you will help to lead me out. When I'm listening to lies, you'll remind me of the truth. And in God's strength, I will do these things for you.

In the world's eyes, redemption looks like individuals triumphing over adversity. But in God's kingdom, it's displayed through a community of limping pilgrims, carrying one another in the light: 'If we walk in the light, as he is in the light, we have fellowship with one another, and the blood of Jesus . . . purifies us from all sin' (1 John 1:7).

Reviewing the day

We started our day alone in the dark. We finish it as a community, knit together in love. So what happens next?

If this were a Hollywood movie, we'd laugh about our struggles and say, 'Thank goodness they're behind us. Thank God we're fixed . . .'. We'd step into eternal sunshine, knowing that the darkness is ended. That would be such a great ending, wouldn't it?

But it's not this one. At least, not quite yet.

A time *is* coming when there'll be no more darkness. Everything will be made new (Matthew 19:28), and every part of us will be healed and made whole. When Jesus returns, there will be no more suffering:

Our wounds will be healed.
Our struggles will be redeemed.
Our relationships will be made perfect.
Our world will be restored.

This is the future, and it's coming soon. However, for a little while longer, we wait. We remember that we belong to the day and not the night (1 Thessalonians 5:5). And in the light of God's presence, we keep walking.

So, as we press forwards, let's recap on where we've been.

When it comes to mental and spiritual health, we're all in the same boat. We *all* wrestle with hunger, anxiety, control, shame, anger and despair. We're all sinners and we're all sick. Since Adam and Eve every part of us is broken. We try to fix ourselves, but we're lost in the dark.

Jesus sees our suffering and our sin. Yet he takes a surprising approach to the darkness. Instead of avoiding it, or lifting us out, he enters it himself. At the cross he bears it. And as he rises from the grave, he defeats it and brings us into a kingdom of light (Colossians 1:13).

When we follow Jesus, we take on his name and are brought into God's family. But this isn't just a one-off event (see Luke 9:23). It's a lifelong process of giving our hearts and minds and bodies and relationships to him. As with every marriage, it takes time to grow into our new identity. This means we'll sometimes forget who we are and fall into old patterns. However, when we stumble, we go back to the cross. Every day we will fall, but every day he will give us new strength.

The pattern of the Christian life is struggle now, celebrations later; the darkness of the cross, then the light of resurrection. Darkness is not a detour. We journey through 'the valley of the shadow', knowing that this is the path and none of our sufferings is wasted. As Sam puts it in *The Two Towers*,

> It's like in the great stories, Mr. Frodo, the ones that really mattered. Full of darkness and danger they were, and sometimes you didn't want to know the end because how

could the end be happy? How could the world go back
to the way it was when so much bad had happened? But
in the end, it's only a passing thing this shadow, even
darkness must pass. A new day will come, and when the
sun shines it'll shine out the clearer.[1]

I don't know what you're facing right now or how hard it
is for you to keep walking. I don't know where you've come
from or what the future will bring. But I do know this:
Christ has overcome the dark and he is at work *in* our mess.
God is using this 'passing shadow', to bring an even
brighter glory.

Right now our relationship with Jesus is like seeing our
lover reflected in a grubby mirror, but then it will be 'face
to face' (1 Corinthians 13:12). Right now it's like the
darkest night, but then it will be eternal dawn (2 Peter
1:19). Right now it's like the pains of childbearing, but
then it will be like the joy of a newborn child (Romans
8:22). Right now we're like acorns – but we're going to be
oaks! (Isaiah 61:3).

With God as our Father, Jesus as our Brother, the Spirit
as our Helper and the church as our family, none of us is
ever alone in the dark. So, arm in arm, let's keep going.

It's a new day and, together, we can walk in the light.

Wait for the LORD;
   be strong and take heart
   and wait for the LORD.
(Psalm 27:14)

Appendix
Advice on specific issues

Eating disorders

Offering support
- Express concern, but prepare for denial, tears and anger. Be gentle but firm, and try to give specific examples, for instance 'I've noticed you go to the toilet after every meal and your face looks puffy and red.'
- If you think your loved one is in immediate danger, then get help straight away.
- Focus on feelings and relationships, not on weight and food, and try not to comment on how the sufferer looks. Remember that most EDs are not immediately obvious.
- Don't try to be a therapist or to cope alone. Where possible, work with others: families, pastors, friends and professionals.

- Move forward. The goal is not necessarily to get the old person back to where he or she was, especially if the individual was in unhealthy patterns. Pray for a new vision of what can be, and view recovery not as a detour, but as part of the process.
- Be patient, as recovery can be a long process.
- Support the whole family, for example by taking siblings out or meeting up with parents.

At meal times:

- Don't offer too much choice: For example, instead of asking, 'Would you like a yogurt?', ask instead, 'What flavour yogurt would you like?'
- Stick to meal plans and agreed routines. It helps sufferers to know in advance what they're eating and where. However, discourage the sufferer from further involvement in meal planning or preparation (especially in the early stages of recovery).
- Don't bribe, don't blackmail and don't renegotiate – especially at mealtimes.
- Offer lots of encouragement and reassurance: 'You're doing really well. I can see this is hard, but I'm so proud of you.'
- If you notice unusual behaviour, then gently raise it along with how the sufferer feels. For example, 'I can see you're struggling with your meat and hiding it under your vegetables. Can you talk to me about why that's hard?'
- Provide distractions after meals, such as soothing music, journaling, arts and crafts, deep breathing, board games or watching a film.[1]

If you suspect your child has an eating disorder:

- Talk to them. For example, 'I've noticed that you're quieter than usual and you haven't been eating lunch. Can we talk about how you're feeling?'
- Don't blame yourself. Focus on what you can do and on opening up conversation.
- Make an appointment with your GP and explain your concerns. When did the behaviours start? What sort of physical and emotional changes have you noticed? How does your child talk about his or her body? Have others commented, such as teachers or friends?
- Work as a family team. Be consistent, support each other and be prepared for lies and emotional outbursts.
- Suggest how others can pray or help. They may want to, but need direction on how to do so.
- Emphasize internal qualities such as kindness. Talk about TV and media representations of looks and images. Compare these to the Bible's focus on character and love for the Lord.
- Monitor Internet use. Be aware of pro-eating disorder websites under the tags 'pro-ana' (anorexia) or 'pro-mia' (bulimia).
- Teach about the importance of emotions, and how to manage them. Explain that 'fat' isn't a feeling, but a word that can be used to hide how we really feel. Talk about the difference between physical and emotional hunger and how they can get mixed up. Physical hunger is when our tummies need food; emotional hunger is when we need to share our feelings. Explain that feelings (even uncomfortable ones) are healthy and they don't need to be stuffed, hidden or starved.

- Continue to include your child in family activities and social arrangements (even if he or she doesn't join in).

Don't feel ashamed or think that your family is more broken than anyone else's because your sibling has an eating disorder. There is no perfect family. God can draw you closer to him and each other through your troubles.

If you are a sibling, be a friend to your sister/brother with an eating disorder. They get challenged all the time by parents. Sometimes it is most loving to just do normal things. We all need a soft place to land (grace). No-one wants to be seen as just a case that needs fixing. Underneath it all they are still the same person whom you knew when they were well.

See also *Eating Disorders: Helping Your Child Recover*, published by B-eat, www.b-eat.co.uk/Shop/Bookshop.

Understanding OCD

Know the facts:

1. You can't always spot someone with OCD. Often it's internal, for example worrying if you're going to harm someone or write something blasphemous.
2. It's not necessarily about being super-organized or tidy. Up to two-thirds of sufferers are also hoarders, which can be the opposite of neat.
3. It's not caused by religion. Sufferers may be attracted to rituals, but the gospel offers hope, grace and freedom from works.

ADVICE ON SPECIFIC ISSUES

4. OCD is a mental illness, not a catch-all phrase for having quirks or wanting things a certain way.
5. OCD is not just an issue for adults. It's estimated that at least one in every 100 children and teens has OCD.[2]
6. OCD can be managed and often responds to treatment, such as CBT (cognitive behavioural therapy).
7. Sufferers are rarely dangerous to themselves or others. They don't carry out their thoughts or fears – in fact, their obsession is with preventing them.

Offering support

- Encourage sufferers to seek help and to keep taking medication, if appropriate.
- Look out for warning signs, for example seeking reassurance, doing things over and over, irritability/ indecisiveness, extreme reactions to minor things, spending a long time doing activities/being late, taking longer than usual over small tasks.
- Don't provide reassurance about specific obsessions, or support sufferers in their rituals. For example, if they repeatedly ask, 'Are you sure I turned the oven off?', don't keep saying 'yes'. It's natural to want to help, but this can reinforce their behaviour, protect them from its negative effects and discourage them from seeking treatment. Instead, the goal is to teach sufferers to sit with their anxiety and to allow it to pass, not to rely on you to manage it.
- Be calm and accepting. Disturbing thoughts or impulses can be part of the condition, and sufferers need to know that you are not judging them.

- Try to keep life as normal as possible, for example by containing routines to one room rather than the whole house. Don't let OCD dominate conversations, and set limits on discussions about specific worries.
- Celebrate little changes, such as checking twice that the doors are locked instead of three times. These might seem small, but to the sufferer they're big, and your encouragement is a powerful motivator.
- If you're a preacher, try to be sensitive to sufferers. Remind them that sin is slavery as well as a choice, discourage them from too much self-analysis, and preach grace: that Jesus deals with our sin, not us.

Sexual abuse

Know the facts:

- Sexual abuse *does not* necessarily involve penetration or physical harm.
- Around 30–40% of victims are abused by family members. Half have been abused by someone outside the immediate family, whom they know and trust.
- Secrecy and denial are common, which makes it difficult to estimate how many are affected. More than 30% of children never tell anyone about their abuse. Almost 80% initially deny it and don't want to disclose anything. Of those who do, more than 20% will later deny it ever happened.[3]
- Sexual abuse affects every aspect of a person's life. This may include undiagnosed mental health issues or physical problems like stomach cramps.

- Survivors may blame God for not stopping the abuse, especially if clergy members are implicated. If the abuser was an older man, this can translate into a negative view of fatherhood and authority. If the abuser was an older woman, this can have a similarly negative impact on the victim's understanding of motherhood/femininity.
- Survivors may feel unable to go to their families for support, especially if relatives are implicated. However, the family's response to abuse is a significant factor in how they will cope long term. If family members blame the victim or cover up the abuse, it feels like a double betrayal.
- Older victims may assume responsibility for their abuse, particularly when they know the perpetrator (which is usually the case). This is complicated by the fact that our bodies are programmed to respond positively to sexual stimulation, even when it's exploitative.

Offering support
- Stay calm, listen and reassure the person that you believe them.
- Have clear structures for reporting and dealing with abuse, including a child protection officer and pastoral team, with links to specialist support networks.
- Be understanding of the strategies that survivors may be using to cope. It is common for those who have been sexually abused to struggle with mental health issues such as self-harm and depression (and for these issues to mask their abuse). They may also have addictions, particularly relating to the body and self-nurture, such as sex and food:

I grew up with domestic violence and a history of physical and sexual abuse . . . as a kid I shut down all my emotions as a way to cope . . . I needed a way to switch it all off and make myself like stone again. Self-harm fulfilled that need pretty effectively for a while.

- Provide a safe space for survivors to process their emotions, and allow them to be open and honest about how they feel (including their anger towards God). Avoid giving pat answers.
- Don't rush survivors through recovery. Addressing the issues (and considerations of forgiveness) takes time. Be aware of the impact that this has on existing relationships, especially with family members or others who were involved.
- Be patient. Survivors may seek to regain control over their circumstances or other people, and they can be highly demanding of themselves and others. They may find it difficult to build relationships/trust and to manage their emotions – perhaps suppressing them in unhealthy ways or overreacting to trivial incidents.
- Refer survivors to outside help if they want it.

Self-harm

Offering support
- Acknowledge your feelings, even if they're mixed, and try not to transfer your emotions to the sufferer.
- Stay calm and try not to judge. Remember that you're dealing with a mental illness, and that sufferers are probably already condemning themselves.

- Offer support instead of ultimatums. Express your concern and let the person know that you're available if he or she wants to talk.
- Encourage communication and build trust. If the individual hasn't told you about the self-harming, bring up the subject in a caring, non-confrontational way. For example, 'I've noticed injuries on your body, and I want to understand what you're going through.' Encourage openness about struggles, but not fascination with the acts themselves.
- Know your limits. Accept that being involved with someone who self-harms can be very stressful. Work out what level of support you can offer, and don't try to cope alone.
- Be practical. You can't stop someone self-harming, but you can check that the wounds are being treated and offer to take the sufferer to the GP if these seem serious or become infected. This can protect against excessive scarring or hidden damage such as unrepaired tendons.
- Encourage sufferers to include Jesus in their struggles by praying together or alone. Remind sufferers that they are not condemned, but that Jesus loves them and is for them. This remains true, even when they don't feel it.

Depression

Signs to watch out for
The sufferer

- seems uncharacteristically sad, irritable, short-tempered, critical or moody. Talks about feeling

'helpless' or 'hopeless', and lacks interest in things he or she used to enjoy, like work, hobbies, and so on.
- withdraws from friends, family and other social activities.
- sleeps less or is oversleeping.
- eats more or less than usual, and may have gained or lost weight.
- may be indecisive, forgetful, disorganized or seem detached from reality.
- relies on alcohol, sleeping tablets, drugs or prescription medications.

Offering support
- Invite sufferers out for gentle activities in low-stress locations (e.g. exercise can help) and provide practical help with shopping, chores, and so on. Be prepared to meet them in their own home or where they feel most secure, and be 'easy company' (e.g. watch a DVD together).
- Help them to attend appointments and to keep taking their medication (if appropriate).
- Don't assume that it's a spiritual issue:

> It really distresses me when the message given is: 'Sort your relationship out with God and your mental health issues will go away.' While I truly believe that God is sovereign and that he can heal mental health difficulties, he often doesn't. While there can be spiritual aspects to mental health (particularly in how we respond to the illnesses), we need to remember to offer support and understanding across all aspects.
>
> [In church] there seem to be two approaches: the 'pray-and-it'll-be-all-better camp', which is a total nightmare, since

a) it's not true, and b) it makes feelings of failure even worse. The opposite approach – 'Let me stand with you' – has been the biggest blessing ever.

- Empathize and care, but beware of trying to fix or silence others so that you can feel better. Sometimes God works not by removing distress, but by revealing himself in the midst of it.
- Ask questions if you think someone is struggling, but don't force them to talk.
- Be alert to signs that sufferers are getting worse or considering suicide. These signs can include talking about suicide or seeming preoccupied with dying; acting in dangerous and self-destructive ways; saying goodbye or seeming to tie up life affairs; stockpiling pills, and so on; or suddenly appearing calm after feeling very low. Talk to them and seek help from their GP/care team. Say, 'I'm worried about you. You seem to be losing hope. Are you thinking of doing harm to yourself?' Stay calm and listen.
- Remind sufferers that depression does *not* make them a bad Christian or person. Tell them why they are precious to you and to God. And be open to God teaching you through them – he works through struggling people.

Further help

Note: The author and publisher have made every effort to ensure that the external website and email addresses included in this book are correct and up to date at the time of going to press. The author and publisher are not responsible for the content, quality or continuing accessibility of the sites.

My blog: <http://emmascrivener.net>. Articles and posts on mental health and Christian identity as well as useful links and a contact page.

My book: *A New Name* (IVP, 2012). My testimony, available from good bookshops, or from <http://www. ivpbooks.com>.

What Does the Bible Say about Eating Disorders? (Day One, 2016). A short booklet aimed at both sufferers and carers.

Investigating Christianity

- Three Two One: <http://three-two-one.org>. My
  husband's site – and a great explanation of the gospel.
- Christianity Explored: <http://christianityexplored.
  org>. Includes details of seeker courses running at
  churches in your area.

Eating disorders

- Anorexia and Bulimia Care: <http://www.
  anorexiabulimiacare.co.uk>. Organization run by
  Christians for sufferers, families and carers
  (sufferers' helpline: 01934 710679; parents' helpline:
  01934 71064).
- National Centre for Eating Disorders: <http://www.
  eating-disorders.org.uk>. National network of
  counsellors, including telephone treatment options.
- Beat: <https://www.b-eat.co.uk>. UK charity
  supporting those affected by EDs.
- Men Get Eating Disorders Too: <http://
  mengetedstoo.co.uk>. Run by and for men with
  eating disorders, including their carers and families.
- F.E.A.S.T. (Families Empowered and Supporting
  Treatment of Eating Disorders): <http://www.
  feast-ed.org>. Provides support for parents and carers.

Anxiety

- Anxiety UK: <http://www.anxietyuk.org.uk>. A
  user-led organization for those affected by anxiety
  disorders (0844 477 5774).

- No Panic: <http://wwww.nopanic.org.uk>. Provides support to those suffering from anxiety disorders, as well as families and carers (0808 808 0545).
- Social Anxiety UK: <http://www.social-anxiety.org.uk>. Volunteer-led organization with chat rooms, support/social groups and information on CBT.
- Anxiety No More: <http://www.anxietynomore. co.uk>. Information and advice on all aspects of anxiety and panic.
- Big White Wall: <http://www.bigwhitewall.com>. Aims to improve mental health and emotional well-being.
- Calm Clinic: <http://www.calmclinic.com>. Provides information relating to anxiety, panic disorder, stress and depression.
- No More Panic: <http://www.nomorepanic.co.uk>. Information for sufferers about panic, anxiety, phobias and OCD.
- Patient info: <http://www.patient.co.uk>. Self-help on panic attacks, phobias, anxiety, stress, OCD and relaxation exercises.
- Surgery Door: <http://www.surgerydoor.co.uk>. Self-help for anxiety.

OCD

- OCD UK: <http://www.ocduk.org>. Information for children and adults.
- OCD Action: <http://www.ocdaction.org.uk>. The UK's largest OCD charity.
- Beyond OCD: <http://beyondocd.org/information-for-friends-and-family>. Resources for friends and family.

- <http://beyondocd.org/information-for-clergy/recognizing-and-counseling-people-who-have-scrupulosity>. Resources for clergy.

Perfectionism

- Will van der Hart and Rob Waller, *The Perfectionism Book* (IVP, 2016).

Sexual abuse

- Darkness to Light: <http://www.d2l.org>. Provides training and information on preventing child sexual abuse.
- Dan Allender centre: <http://www.theallendercenter.org/conferences/wounded-heart>. Christian resources, conferences and articles on surviving abuse (based in US). See also *The Wounded Heart: Hope for Adult Victims of Childhood Sexual Abuse* (Tyndale House, 2014), an excellent book and audio CD on dealing with sexual abuse.
- Mind.org: <http://www.mind.org.uk/information-support/guides-to-support-and-services/abuse>. Range of resources/help for all kinds of abuse.
- NSPCC: <http://www.nspcc.org.uk/preventing-abuse/signs-symptoms-effects>. Help for children and adult survivors of childhood abuse.
- The Survivor's Trust: <http://www.thesurvivorstrust.org>. National umbrella agency for over 135 specialist rape, sexual violence and childhood sexual abuse support organizations throughout the UK and Ireland.

- Survivors UK: <http://www.survivorsuk.org>. For male survivors of sexual abuse.
- Victim Support: <http://www.victimsupport.org.uk>. Support for women affected by rape or abuse.

Self-harm

- The Site: <http://www.thesite.org/healthandwellbeing/ mentalhealth/selfharm>. Information and discussion boards.
- Self-injury support: <http://www.selfinjurysupport. org.uk/resources>. Includes a list of resources.
- Self-injury.org: <http://www.self-injury.org>. Christian-based self-injury resources.

Anger

- Association of Biblical Counsellors: <http:// christiancounseling.com/content/understanding- and-redeeming-anger>. A useful article on anger.
- Women's Aid: <http://womensaid.co.uk>. For female victims of domestic violence.
- Mankind Initiative: <http://new.mankind.org.uk>. For men affected by domestic violence.
- Hidden Hurt: <http://hiddenhurt.co.uk>. Domestic abuse information, including help for abusers.
- Blain Nelson's blog: <http://blainn.com>. A former abuser talks about getting help.

Depression

- Families for Depression Awareness: <http://www.familyaware.org>. Helping families to recognize and cope with depression and bipolar disorder.
- Seasonal Affective Disorder Association: <http://www.sada.org.uk>.
- Mind: <http://www.mind.org.uk>. Mental health charity with a range of links and resources.
- MAMuk: <http://meetamumuk.forumotion.co.uk>. Online forum offering support and friendship to all mothers and mothers-to-be.
- Black Dog Institute: <http://www.blackdoginstitute.org.au>. Australian site on mood disorders.
- British Association for Behavioural and Cognitive Therapies: <http://www.babcp.com>. Includes self-help and a list of therapists.
- Undoing Depression: <http://www.undoingdepression.com>. Self-help site.
- Depression Alliance: <http://www.depressionalliance.org>. Includes a 'pen-friend' scheme that puts you in touch with other sufferers.
- Students against Depression: <http://www.studentsagainstdepression.org>. Website for students.
- Quarentia: <http://markmeynell.net/blog/2015/08/black-dog-10-years>. An excellent blog series on depression.

Suicide

- Samaritans: <http://www.samaritans.org>. Twenty-four-hour service, available every day of the year. Email support at jo@samaritans.org.

- Papyrus: <http://www.papyrus-uk.org>. Voluntary organization that supports teenagers and young adults who are feeling suicidal.
- CALM: <http://www.thecalmzone.net>. Includes a support group for young men (0800 58 58 58).
- SOBS (Survivors of Bereavement by Suicide): <http://www.uk-sobs.org.uk>. Support for those aged 18 and over (0844 561 6855).

General mental health

- Mind and Soul: <http://www.mindandsoul.info>. Helpful Christian site with various resources on mental health.
- Mercy Ministries: <http://mercyuk.org>. Provides a free, residential Christian discipleship programme for women aged between 18 and 28, who are struggling with issues such as self-harm, eating disorders or abuse.
- Health Talk: <http://www.healthtalkonline.org>. Video, articles and recordings where people share their experiences, for example with depression. Includes a youth section.
- Patient Info: <http://www.patient.co.uk>. Evidence-based health advice, written by doctors.
- NHS: <http://www.nhs.uk/news>. Health news, including a 'Behind the Headlines' section for those who are interested in major health stories, but unsure of the facts behind them.
- Association of Biblical Counsellors: <https://christiancounseling.com>. Provides resources, training and a list of counsellors.

- British Association for Behavioural and Cognitive Psychotherapies (BACP): <http://www.bacp.com>. To read more on CBT from a Christian perspective: <http://christthetruth.net/2010/05/01/cbt-from-a-christian-perspective>.

Notes

1 Evening

1. A Twitter poem, © Glen Scrivener.
2. Emma Scrivener, *A New Name: Grace and Healing for Anorexia* (IVP, 2012), pp. 111–112.
3. Ibid., p. 66.
4. https://www.b-eat.co.uk/about-beat/media-centre/ information-and-statistics-about-eating-disorders (August 2014). Accessed 20 July 2016.
5. Corrie ten Boom, *Clippings from My Notebook* (Thomas Nelson Inc., 1982).
6. American Psychiatric Association, *Diagnostic and Statistical Manual of Mental Disorders*, 5th edn (American Psychiatric Publishing, 2013).
7. http://www.theguardian.com/society/2013/sep/15/ anxiety-epidemic-gripping-britain (September 2013). Accessed 20 July 2016.
8. Report by the Mental Health Foundation in England (2009), http://www.communitycare.co.uk/2009/04/08/ mental-health-foundation-uk-society-becoming-more-fearful. Accessed 22 August 2016.

9. http://www.ocdeducationstation.org/ocd-facts (August 2014). Accessed 20 July 2016.

10. *A New Name*, p. 139.

11. Interview with Sue Perkins, *The Times Magazine* (9 February 2013).

12. https://www.theguardian.com/media/2015/jul/18/katie-hopkins-jon-ronson-interview (July 2015). Accessed 18 July 2016.

13. See Dan Allender, *The Wounded Heart* (Tyndale House, 2014).

14. http://www.crossrhythms.co.uk/keyquotes/index.php?p=3&cat=23/ (August–December 2014). Accessed 20 July 2016.

15. *A New Name*, p. 67.

16. Unless otherwise listed, source for all statistics: http://www.angermanage.co.uk/data.html (2008). Accessed 22 August 2016.

17. https://www.tuc.org.uk/industrial-issues/workplace-issues/health-and-safety/violence/one-eight-people-experience-violence. Accessed 22 August 2016.

18. Health and Safety Executive, Violence at Work (1995), http://www.hse.gov.uk/pubns/indg69.pdf. Accessed 15 August 2016.

19. http://www.theguardian.com/society/2013/jun/19/anxiety-depression-office-national-statistics (June 2013). Accessed 25 July 2016.

20. http://www.mentalhealth.org.uk/help-information/mental-health-statistics/older-people (2002). Accessed 25 July 2016.

21. http://www.reuters.com/article/us-usa-veterans-suicide-idUSBRE9101E320130202 (February 2013). Accessed 25 July 2016.

22. http://www.samaritans.org/about-us/our-research/facts-and-figures-about-suicide (2015). Accessed 25 July 2016.
23. http://www.telegraph.co.uk/culture/8194587/True-grit-Jeff-Bridges-interview.html (December 2010). Accessed 25 July 2016.
24. *A New Name*, pp. 62, 123.

2 Midnight

1. For more on this, see http://www.three-two-one.org. Accessed 25 July 2016.
2. Martin Waddell, *Can't You Sleep, Little Bear?* (Walker Books, 2005), p. 5.

3 The early hours

1. Timothy Keller, 'The Two Advocates', *Encounters with Jesus: Unexpected Answers to Difficult Questions* (Hodder & Stoughton, 2013), ch. 7.

4 Dawn

1. D. Martyn Lloyd-Jones, *Spiritual Depression: Its Causes and Cure* (Marshall Pickering, 1970), pp. 20–21.
2. Westminster Confession of Faith (1621), chapter 32 (italics mine). See http://www.reformed.org/documents/wcf_with_proofs/index.html. Accessed 16 August 2016.

5 Morning

1. Lizzie Jank, 'A Spirited Rider', http://www.feminagirls.com/2010/08/19/a-spirited-rider.

NOTES TO PAGES 104-166

2. Scott Stossel, *My Age of Anxiety: Fear, Hope, Dread, and the Search for Peace of Mind* (Windmill Books, 2014).
3. John Piper, *Risk Is Right: Better to Lose Your Life than to Waste It* (Crossway, 2013), p. 47.
4. Emma Scrivener, *A New Name: Grace and Healing for Anorexia* (IVP, 2012), p. 134.
5. Steven Levenkron, *Cutting: Understanding and Overcoming Self-Mutilation* (W. W. Norton, 1998), p. 80.
6. Philip Yancey, *What's So Amazing about Grace?* (Zondervan, 1997), p. 99.
7. Timothy Keller, *The Grieving Sisters*, The Encounters with Jesus Series, 3 (Hodder & Stoughton, 2013).

6 Afternoon

1. Caitlin Moran, *Moranifesto* (Ebury Press, 2016), pp. 433–434.
2. http://www.mindandsoul.info/Groups/250563/Mind_and_Soul/Resources/Topics/Medication/Medication.aspx. Accessed 25 July 2016.
3. Report by the Children's Commissioner for England (2015). See http://www.thetimes.co.uk/article/nhs-turns-away-children-with-life-threatening-mental-illness-2hnw3gnxj. Accessed June 2016.
4. http://www.independent.co.uk/life-style/health-and-families/health-news/thousands-attempt-suicide-while-on-nhs-waiting-list-for-psychological-help-9734284.html (September 2014). Accessed 10 August 2016.
5. John Stott, *The Radical Disciple: Some Neglected Aspects of Our Calling* (IVP, 2010), p. 110.
6. Taken from entry for 8 July, in Henri J. M. Nouwen, *Bread for the Journey: A Daybook of Wisdom and Faith* (HarperOne, 1985).

7. Dietrich Bonhoeffer, *Life Together: The Classic Exploration of Christian Community* (Harper & Row, 1954), pp. 118–119 (italics mine).

Reviewing the day

1. Screenplay of *The Lord of the Rings: The Two Towers* (New Line Cinema, 2002), http://www.fempiror.com/otherscripts/LordoftheRings2-TTT.pdf, pp. 207–208.

Appendix

1. Source: British Columbia Children's Hospital, 'Meal Support, Introduction for Parents, Friends and Caregivers'; Auckland Eating Disorder Service, booklet for carers (2008).
2. http://www.ocdeducationstation.org/ocd-facts. Accessed 25 July 2016.
3. Darkness to Light: http://oldsite.d2l.org/KnowAbout/statistics_2.asp. Accessed 21 July 2016.